# Anti Inflammatory Cookbook for Easy Recipes

## 2000 Days of Nourishing and Flavourful Recipes for Optimal Health with a 30-day Meal Plan

© 2025 by Shark Publications. All rights reserved.

No part of this publication may be reproduced, distributed, or transmitted in any form or by any means, including photocopying, recording, or other electronic or mechanical methods, without the prior written permission of the publisher, except in the case of brief quotations embodied in critical reviews and specific other noncommercial uses permitted by copyright law.

Library of Congress Cataloging-in-Publication Data
Names: Rocky Hansen, author.
Title: Anti Inflammatory Cookbook for Easy Recipes: 2000 Days of Nourishing and Flavourful Recipes for Optimal Health with a 30-day Meal Plan.
Description: First Edition. | Includes index.
Subjects: Health & Cookbook—Recipes. | Anti Inflammation—Recipes. | Cooking (Natural foods). | Cooking (Oils and fats).

Cover design by [Hollybookstore]
Interior design by [Rocky Hansen]
Photography by [Rocky Hansen]

Printed in [USA]
First Printing, [03,2025]

This book is dedicated to everyone on their journey to health and wellness through the plant based lifestyle. May you find joy, inspiration, and deliciousness on every page.

While the author and publisher have made every effort to ensure the accuracy and completeness of the information conveyed in this book, they assume no responsibility for errors, inaccuracies, omissions, or any inconsistency herein. Any slights of people, places, or organizations are unintentional.

The recipes and content in this book are intended as a helpful guide and should not replace medical, nutritional, or health advice from a professional. Readers are advised to consult a healthcare provider before starting any new diet or exercise program.

# FREE 300+RECIPES & COMPLETE HEALTH GUIDE

Unlock the full power of your healthy-living journey by claiming your FREE "300-Recipe & Complete Health Guide" bundle—a carefully curated treasury of quick, crave-worthy dishes, science-backed wellness tips, and step-by-step meal plans designed to help you nourish your body and reclaim your energy every single day. Just drop your best email in the sign-up box, and you'll instantly receive this digital collection (no strings attached!) so you can start cooking smarter, feeling lighter, and living better—while gaining VIP access to future exclusive recipes, updates, and bonus resources I only share with my inner circle. If you don't receive the email even after signing up, then please check your **SPAM** folder and **promotional** section in your email. If you still don't find it, then please write Hi to **shark.publications@gmail.com** and I will send it to you personally.

**Scan the QR code to get your FREE Meal Prep Guide**

# CONTENTS

- **1** — INTRODUCTION
- **2** — ANTI-INFLAMMATORY SUPERFOODS
- **4** — FOODS TO EAT AND FOODS TO AVOID
- **10** — MEAL PREP

## Breakfast

- **14** — GINGER-PEACH OATMEAL
  ALMOND BUTTER BANANA PANCAKES
- **15** — BLUEBERRY WALNUT YOGURT PARFAIT
  AVOCADO DEVILED EGGS
- **16** — BERRY ALMOND OVERNIGHT OATS
  ZUCCHINI & ONION FRITTATA
- **17** — CUCUMBER AVOCADO TOAST
  QUINOA & BERRY BREAKFAST BOWL
- **18** — PUMPKIN SPICE OATMEAL
  PEAR & WALNUT OATMEAL
- **19** — COCONUT MILK CHIA PUDDING
  CARROT CAKE OATMEAL

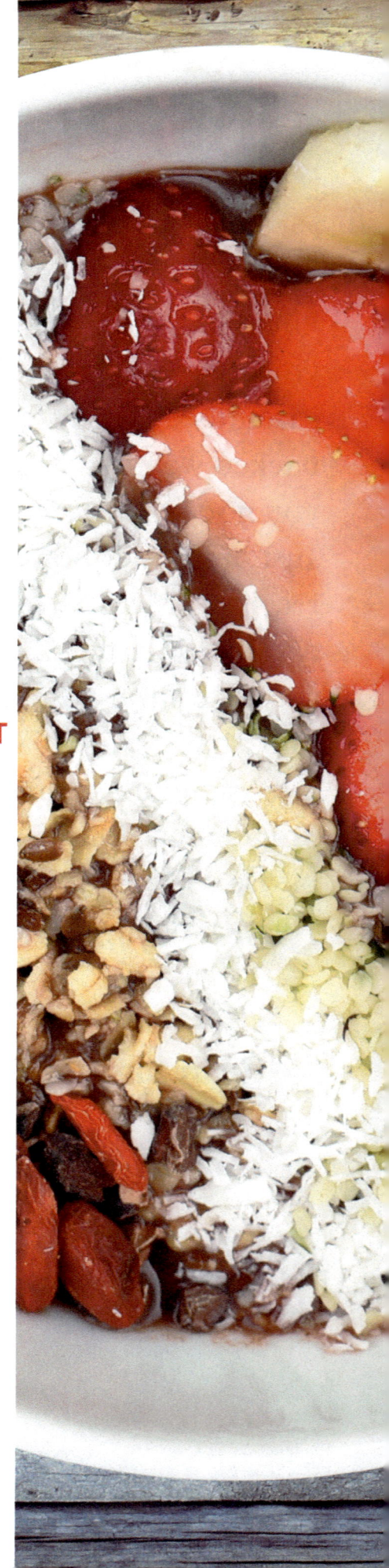

| 20 | **TOFU SCRAMBLE WITH SPINACH** <br> **GINGER PEAR BREAKFAST SALAD** |
|---|---|
| 21 | **SCALLION PANCAKE** <br> **TURMERIC OATS BOWL** |
| 22 | **ANTI-INFLAMMATORY BOWL** <br> **PUMPKIN SEED AND OAT BREAKFAST BARS** |

## SEA FOOD

| 23 | **SALMON SALAD** <br> **SHRIMP FRIED RICE** |
|---|---|
| 24 | **SHRIMP AND GRAPEFRUIT SALAD** <br> **SALMON NIÇOISE SALAD** |
| 25 | **SALMON CURRY RECIPE** <br> **SALMON FISH CAKES** |
| 26 | **TUNA STEAKS WITH MANGO SALSA** <br> **SHRIMP WITH QUINOA** |
| 27 | **TUNA STUFFED AVOCADO RECIPE** <br> **PISTACHIO SALMON** |
| 28 | **COD AND ASPARAGUS** <br> **PRAWN AND BROCCOLI COCONUT CURRY** |
| 29 | **TILAPIA WITH BROCCOLI** <br> **LEMON BASIL SALMON** |
| 30 | **TERIYAKI SALMON WITH MANGO** <br> **SEAFOOD PAELLA** |

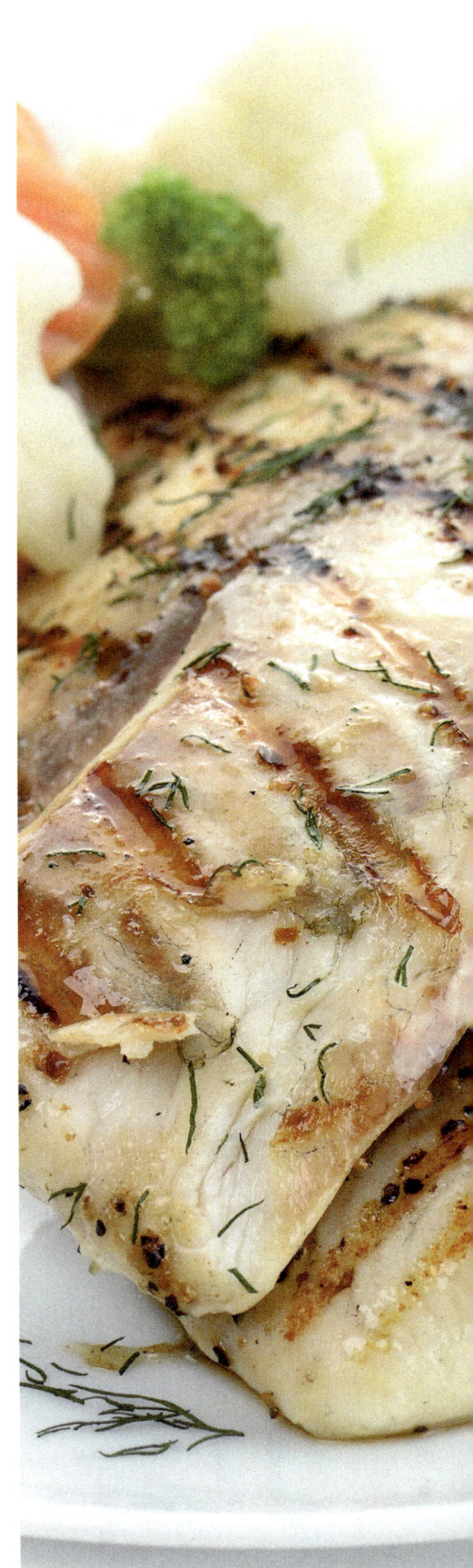

| 31 | **SALMON WITH FENNEL SALAD** <br> **FIERY PRAWNS** |
|---|---|
| 32 | **CREAMY LEEK AND SALMON SOUP** <br> **COCONUT SOUP WITH SHRIMP** |
| 33 | **TUNA AND STRAWBERRY SALAD** <br> **TUNA POKE BOWL RECIPE** |
| 34 | **SALMON WITH CARROTS AND BROCCOLI** <br> **CAJUN JUMBO SHRIMP** |
| 35 | **TUNA AND WHITE BEAN SALAD** <br> **PAN-SEARED TUNA STEAKS** |
| 36 | **SALMON AND AVOCADO TOAST** <br> **WALNUT-CRUSTED SALMON** |

## VEGETARIAN

| 37 | **FETA, AND OLIVE SALAD** <br> **AVOCADO AND CHICKPEA SANDWICH** |
|---|---|
| 38 | **VEGAN BLACK BEAN BURGERS** <br> **CAULIFLOWER TACOS** |
| 39 | **MEDITERRANEAN QUINOA SALAD** <br> **MUSHROOM STROGANOFF** |
| 40 | **BUTTERNUT SQUASH RISOTTO** <br> **VEGAN SHEPHERD'S PIE** |

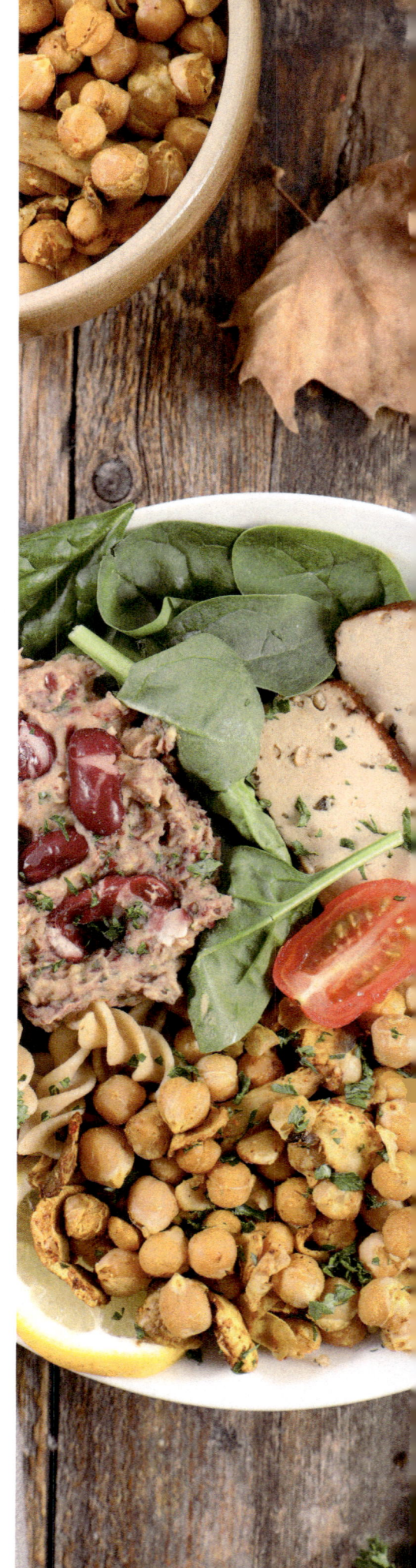

| | |
|---|---|
| **41** | **PROTEIN-PACKED TOFU SCRAMBLE** <br> **CHICKPEA AND AVOCADO WRAP** |
| **42** | **ROASTED VEGGIE AND FARRO BOWL** <br> **ROASTED CAULIFLOWER SALAD** |
| **43** | **AVOCADO AND WHITE BEAN SALAD** <br> **SWEET POTATO & BLACK BEAN BOWL** |
| **44** | **LENTIL & CARROT SALAD** <br> **ASIAN CABBAGE AND EDAMAME SALAD** |
| **45** | **SPROUTS AND WALNUT SALAD** <br> **CABBAGE AND CHICKPEA SALAD** |
| **46** | **MUSHROOM & SPINACH QUINOA PILAF** <br> **SWEET POTATO AND BLACK BEANENCHILADA** |
| **47** | **ZUCCHINI NOODLE PAD THAI** <br> **SWEET POTATO AND KALE TACOS** |
| **48** | **CREAMY SPINACH & ARTICHOKE PASTA** <br> **PUMPKIN AND SPINACH CURRY** |
| **49** | **CAULIFLOWER RICE & BLACK BEAN BOWL** <br> **MOROCCAN CHICKPEA SOUP** |
| **50** | **MUSHROOM RISOTTO** <br> **VEGAN SPAGHETTI CARBONARA** |
| **51** | **ZUCCHINI NOODLE WITH ALMOND BUTTER** <br> **CASHEW ALFREDO PASTA** |

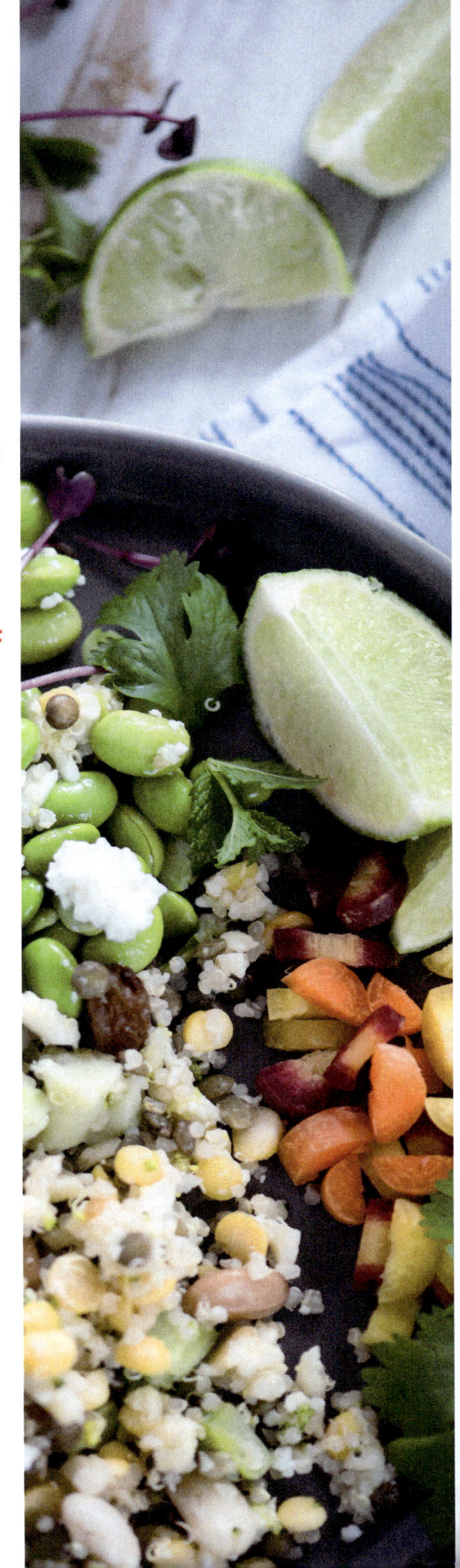

## POULTRY

**52** — TURKEY PATTIES / ROASTED CHICKEN THIGHS

**53** — ASIAN SOUP WITH CHICKEN MEATBALLS / CHICKEN BULGOGI

**54** — CHICKEN HASH RECIPE / COCONUT CHICKEN TENDERS

**55** — EASY COCONUT CHICKEN / EASY CHICKEN + SPINACH

**56** — MANGO AND GRILLED CHICKEN SALAD / CHAYOTE CHICKEN NOODLE SOUP

**57** — POMEGRANATE CHICKEN SALAD / MARINATED GRILLED CHICKEN

**58** — HERBED TURKEY AND VEGETABLE SOUP / JAMAICAN CHICKEN FAJITAS

**59** — CHICKEN SOUP / CURRIED LENTIL CHICKEN SOUP

**60** — GRILLED CHICKEN AND QUINOA SALAD / TURKEY AND SPINACH SWEET POTATOES

**61** — CHICKEN AND BROCCOLI STIR-FRY / TURMERIC CHICKEN WITH VEGETABLES

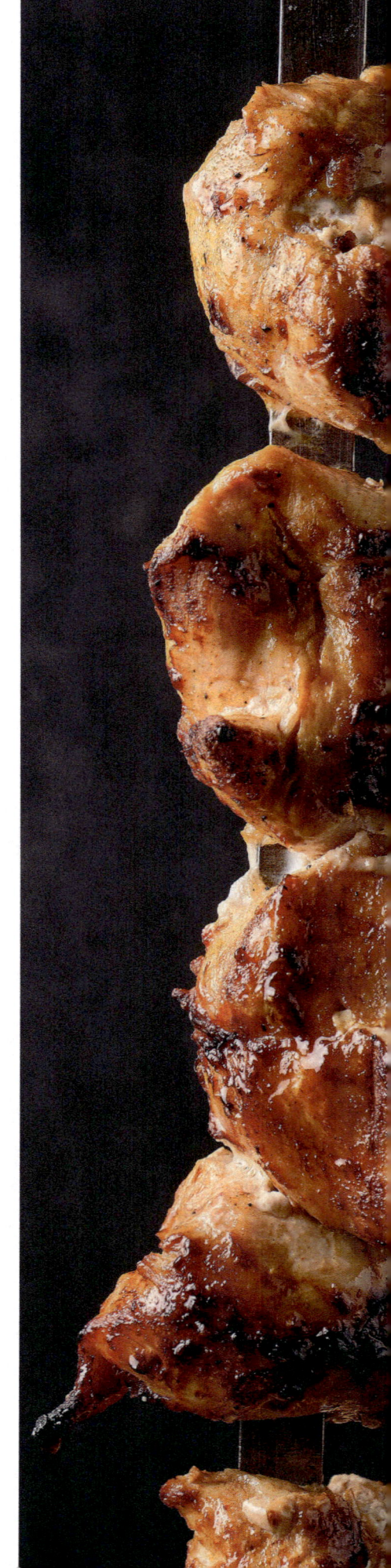

# DESSERTS

**62** — SUMMER BERRY TART / GREEN TEA CHIA PUDDING

**63** — CHIA SEED AND BLUEBERRY PUDDING / RASPBERRY COCONUT BARS

**64** — ZUCCHINI BROWNIES / BAKED PEARS WITH WALNUTS AND HONEY

**65** — MATCHA GREEN TEA ICE CREAM / BLUEBERRY AND LEMON MUFFINS

**66** — CARROT CAKE BITES / WALNUT AND OAT CLUSTERS

**67** — GINGER PEACH SORBET / COCONUT TURMERIC CHIA PUDDING

**68** — CHIA SEED PUDDING / OATMEAL AND BANANA COOKIES

**69** — BERRY SORBET / ALMOND AND DATE TRUFFLES

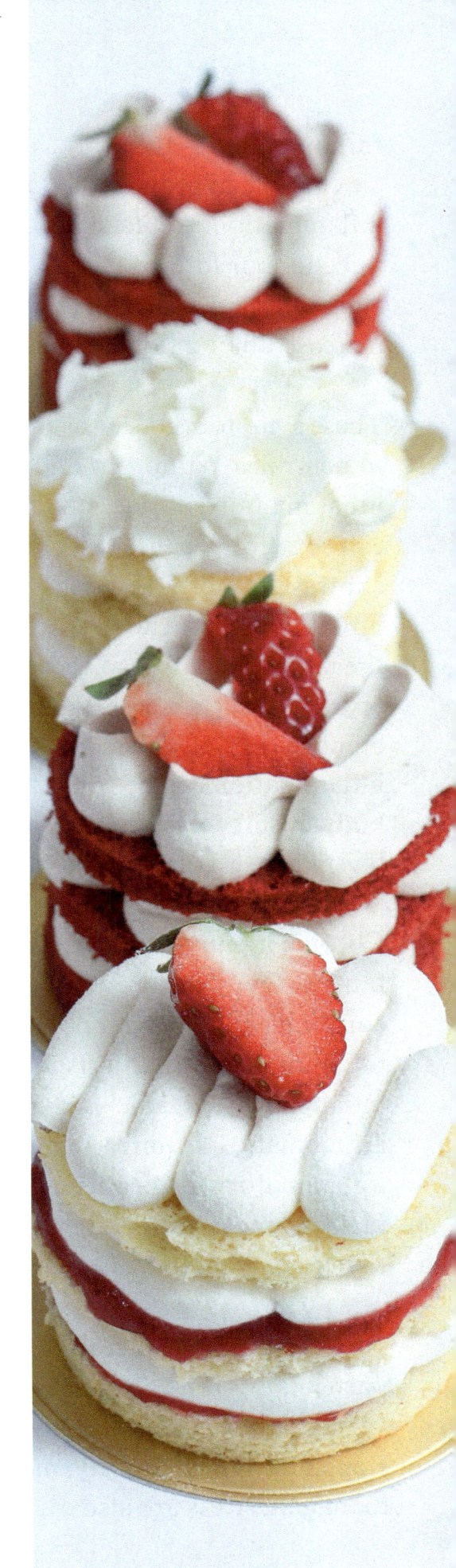

# Introduction

Inflammation is the body's immune response to injury, infection, or irritation, playing a crucial role in healing and defense. It occurs in two primary forms: acute and chronic inflammation. Acute inflammation is a rapid, short-term response to physical injury, infection, or foreign invaders. It starts quickly, often within minutes or hours, and eliminates harmful agents while initiating tissue repair. This response is marked by increased blood flow, redness, swelling, heat, and sometimes pain or loss of function.

These symptoms occur as immune cells, mainly white blood cells, rush to the affected area to neutralize pathogens and clear damaged tissue. Once the threat is eliminated, inflammation subsides, and healing begins. While generally beneficial, acute inflammation can sometimes cause discomfort and requires management. Chronic inflammation, in contrast, is a prolonged immune response lasting months or even years. Unlike acute inflammation, it can persist without an apparent injury or infection or continue even after the initial cause is resolved. It is often associated with severe health conditions, including arthritis, heart disease, diabetes, and certain cancers. This prolonged immune activity can damage the body's tissues, increasing the risk of long-term health complications. Chronic inflammation can be triggered by persistent infections, autoimmune disorders (where the body mistakenly attacks healthy cells), prolonged exposure to environmental irritants, and lifestyle factors like obesity, smoking, and chronic stress.

Chronic inflammation has fewer symptoms than acute inflammation, including persistent fatigue, fever, rashes, and pain. Over time, it can lead to significant tissue damage, contributing to the development of severe diseases. Beyond physical health, chronic inflammation also affects mental well-being. Research links it to depression and anxiety, as inflammatory chemicals can influence brain function, mood, and behavior. Managing inflammation requires a combination of medical treatment and lifestyle changes. Anti-inflammatory medications can help reduce symptoms, while lifestyle adjustments—such as maintaining a healthy diet, managing stress, and avoiding smoking—can play a crucial role in reducing inflammation and supporting overall health.

However, lifestyle factors play a significant role in managing inflammation. Diet, in particular, is crucial; consuming a diet rich in anti-inflammatory foods like fruits, vegetables, whole grains, and omega-3 fatty acids can help reduce inflammation levels. Regular physical activity, maintaining a healthy weight, getting enough sleep, and managing stress are also essential for controlling inflammation.

# Anti-Inflammatory Superfoods

**Antioxidant-Rich Fruits and Vegetables**

Fruits and vegetables are rich in antioxidants that combat inflammation. Blueberries and blackberries contain anthocyanins, while carrots and sweet potatoes provide beta-carotene, which supports immunity. Leafy greens like spinach and Swiss chard offer vitamins E and C and magnesium, further reducing inflammation. Citrus fruits, packed with vitamin C, enhance immune function. Eating a variety of colorful produce maximizes these benefits.

**Cruciferous Vegetables and Sulforaphane**

Broccoli, cauliflower, brussels sprouts, cabbage, and kale are rich in fiber, vitamins, and sulforaphane, a powerful anti-inflammatory compound. Sulforaphane blocks enzymes that trigger inflammation, while fiber supports gut health. To boost its effects, chop these veggies and let them sit before cooking, or eat them raw for maximum benefits.

**Berries and Their Flavonoid Power**

Berries are among the most potent anti-inflammatory fruits. Strawberries, raspberries, blueberries, goji, and acai berries are rich in flavonoids, compounds known for their powerful health benefits. Blueberries, in particular, contain anthocyanins, which combat oxidative stress and inflammation. Regular berry consumption has been linked to lower inflammatory markers. These versatile fruits can be enjoyed in smoothies, salads, and desserts, making them an easy and delicious way to support overall health.

**The Wonders of Omega-3 Fatty Acids**

Omega-3 fatty acids, found in fish, nuts, and seeds, are essential fats with potent anti-inflammatory properties. Fish like salmon, mackerel, sardines, and herring provide EPA and DHA, which support cell membrane health and reduce inflammation. Algal oil is an excellent DHA source for vegetarians and vegans. Fish oil or algal oil supplements can help those with limited dietary intake. Balancing omega-3 and omega-6 intake is crucial. While omega-6 fats are necessary, modern diets often favor them because vegetable oils in processed foods promote inflammation.

To optimize health, increase omega-3-rich whole foods while minimizing excessive omega-6 sources. This balance enhances the anti-inflammatory benefits of omega-3s, supporting long-term well-being. Choosing olive or avocado oil instead of soybean or corn oil can significantly impact your diet. Additionally, being conscious of the source of your foods, reading labels, and making informed choices can play a pivotal role in this balance.

**Whole Grains, Fiber, and Anti-Inflammation**

Unlike refined grains, whole grains like quinoa, oats, and brown rice retain fiber-rich bran, making them powerful anti-inflammatory foods. Their fiber supports gut health, stabilizes blood sugar, and lowers systemic inflammation. Regular consumption promotes heart health, digestion, and weight management. Simple swaps like choosing whole grains over refined ones can enhance overall well-being.

**Anti-Inflammatory Herbs and Spices**

Turmeric, rich in curcumin, reduces inflammation, especially when paired with black pepper for better absorption. Ginger, known for its gingerols, helps combat inflammation and digestive issues. Garlic's sulfur compounds, along with polyphenol-rich herbs like rosemary and oregano, reduce inflammation and boost overall health.

**Lean Proteins and Plant-Based Alternatives**

Fatty fish like salmon and sardines provide omega-3s that counteract inflammation. Plant-based proteins, including lentils, chickpeas, tofu, nuts, and seeds, offer fiber, antioxidants, and beneficial fats. A balanced intake of these proteins supports a healthier, anti-inflammatory diet.

# Foods to eat and foods to avoid

Managing inflammation through diet involves a thoughtful balance of foods, including those that have anti-inflammatory benefits and those that should be avoided because they can exacerbate inflammatory processes.

**Emphasizing Anti-Inflammatory Foods:**

- **Fruits and vegetables:** Various fruits and vegetables should form the foundation of an anti-inflammatory diet. They are packed with vitamins, minerals, fiber, and antioxidants, which help dampen inflammatory processes.

A list of fruits and vegetables that are known for their anti-inflammatory properties:

## Fruits:

- **Berries:** Blueberries, strawberries, raspberries, and blackberries are rich in antioxidants and vitamins.
- **Cherries:** Especially tart cherries are known for their anti-inflammatory effects.
- **Oranges:** High in vitamin C and antioxidants.
- **Grapes:** Contain antioxidants such as resveratrol and flavonoids.
- **Pineapple:** Contains bromelain, an enzyme that may reduce inflammation.
- **Pomegranates:** Rich in antioxidants and flavonoids.
- **Apples:** High in fiber and anti-inflammatory polyphenols.
- **Bananas:** Rich in potassium and magnesium.
- **Kiwi:** High in vitamin C and antioxidants.
- **Papaya:** It contains papain, an enzyme that can help reduce inflammation.
- **Mangoes:** Packed with polyphenols that have anti-inflammatory properties.
- **Watermelon:** Contains lycopene and vitamin C.
- **Grapefruit:** High in vitamin C and antioxidants.

- **Olives and Olive Oil:** High in oleic acid and antioxidants.
- **Black Currants:** High in antioxidants and vitamin C.
- **Plums:** Contain antioxidants and anti-inflammatory agents.
- **Apricots:** Rich in vitamins and flavonoids that can reduce inflammation.
- **Lemons and Limes:** High in vitamin C and antioxidants.
- **Nectarines:** Packed with bioactive compounds, vitamins, and minerals.
- **Cranberries:** Known for their anti-inflammatory properties.
- **Persimmons:** Contain flavonoids and antioxidants.
- **Dragon Fruit:** High in vitamin C, fiber, and antioxidants.

## Vegetables:

- **Leafy Greens:** Spinach, kale, and Swiss chard contain anti-inflammatory flavonoids and antioxidants.
- **Broccoli:** High in sulforaphane, an antioxidant with anti-inflammatory effects.
- **Beets:** Contain betalain, an anti-inflammatory compound.
- **Carrots:** High in beta-carotene and fiber.
- **Brussels Sprouts:** Rich in antioxidants.
- **Cauliflower:** Like broccoli, it's high in antioxidants and beneficial compounds.
- **Asparagus:** High in folate and vitamins, with anti-inflammatory effects.
- **Seaweed:** Rich in omega-3 fatty acids and bioactive compounds.
- **Mushrooms:** Shiitake, especially, are rich in selenium, copper, and all B vitamins.
- **Celery:** Contains luteolin, an antioxidant that reduces inflammation.
- **Artichokes:** High in fiber, inulin, and antioxidants.
- **Kale:** Extremely rich in vitamins K, A, C.

## Grains

- **Brown Rice:** Rich in fiber and selenium, brown rice can help reduce inflammation associated with chronic diseases.

- **Whole Wheat:** Contains fiber, phytonutrients, and antioxidants that may help reduce inflammation.

- **Oats:** Oats are high in beta-glucan, a soluble fiber that can lower inflammation and improve insulin resistance.

- **Barley:** Rich in beta-glucan and antioxidants, barley can help lower inflammation and improve heart health.

- **Quinoa:** High in protein, fiber, and antioxidants.

- **Buckwheat:** High in rutin and other antioxidants.

- **Millet:** Rich in magnesium, which can help lower inflammation and improve insulin response.

## Omega-3-Rich Foods

- **Fatty Fish:** Salmon, mackerel, sardines, trout, and herring are excellent sources of EPA and DHA, two potent omega-3 fatty acids.

- **Chia Seeds:** These tiny seeds are rich in omega-3s, fiber, and protein.

- **Flaxseeds:** Both flaxseeds and flaxseed oil are high in ALA, a plant-based omega-3 fatty acid.

## Nuts

- **Walnuts:** High in omega-3 ALA and antioxidants.

- **Almonds:** Rich in vitamin E, magnesium, and healthy fats.

- **Pistachios:** Rich in healthy fats, fiber, and antioxidants.

- **Pecans:** High in magnesium and antioxidants.

- **Brazil Nuts:** Rich in selenium.

- **Hazelnuts:** They contain high levels of healthy fats and vitamin E.

- **Macadamia Nuts:** They contain monounsaturated fats that have anti-inflammatory effects.

## Seeds

- **Chia Seeds:** Packed with omega-3 fatty acids and fiber.
- **Flaxseeds:** High in omega-3 ALA and lignans.
- **Hemp Seeds:** They provide a good balance of omega-3 and omega-6 fatty acids.
- **Pumpkin Seeds:** They are rich in magnesium.
- **Sunflower Seeds:** High in vitamin E.
- **Sesame Seeds:** Rich in copper, a mineral known for its anti-inflammatory abilities.
- **Quinoa Seeds:** While technically a seed, quinoa is high in protein, fiber, and anti-inflammatory phytonutrients.

## Herbs and Spices:

- **Turmeric:** Contains curcumin, a compound with potent anti-inflammatory and antioxidant properties.
- **Ginger:** Gingerol is a substance with powerful anti-inflammatory and antioxidant effects.
- **Cinnamon:** Known for its anti-inflammatory, antioxidant, and antimicrobial properties.
- **Garlic:** Contains allicin and sulphur compounds that have anti-inflammatory effects.
- **Cayenne Pepper:** Contains capsaicin, which is known to reduce inflammation.
- **Black Pepper:** Piperine, a compound in black pepper, can enhance the absorption of other anti-inflammatory compounds, particularly curcumin.
- **Cloves:** Rich in antioxidants and eugenol, cloves have potent anti-inflammatory properties.
- **Rosemary:** Contains Rosmarinus acid and other anti-inflammatory compounds.
- **Basil:** Offers anti-inflammatory and antibacterial benefits.
- **Oregano:** Contains compounds like carvacrol and thymol, which have anti-inflammatory effects.
- **Thyme:** Rich in anti-inflammatory compounds and beneficial for respiratory and immune health.

- **Fennel Seeds:** Have anti-inflammatory and antioxidant properties.

- **Cardamom:** Known for its antioxidant and anti-inflammatory properties.

- **Coriander:** Contains anti-inflammatory and digestive properties.

- **Dill:** Contains antioxidants and compounds that can help reduce inflammation.

- **Mint:** Known for its soothing properties, mint can help reduce inflammation, particularly in the gastrointestinal tract.

- **Parsley:** Rich in vitamins and flavonoids that have anti-inflammatory effects.

- **Cumin:** Has several anti-inflammatory and antioxidant properties.

- **Nutmeg:** Contains anti-inflammatory compounds that can be beneficial in reducing inflammation.

- **Saffron:** Known for its unique compounds that can help reduce inflammation and oxidative stress.

- **Mustard Seed:** Contains compounds that have anti-inflammatory and pain-relieving properties.

- **Fenugreek:** Known for its anti-inflammatory, antioxidant, and digestive properties.

- **Holy Basil (Tulsi):** Distinct from regular basil, it has potent anti-inflammatory and antioxidant effects.

- **Bay Leaves:** Often used in cooking, they contain compounds with anti-inflammatory properties.

# AVOID

## Fat and Oils

- **Butter**
- **Lard**
- **Margarine**

## Grains

- **All refined grains** (e.g., white bread, white pasta, white rice)

- **Packaged, processed grain-based snacks and desserts** (e.g., biscuits, cakes, cereals, cookies, crackers, muffins)

## Others

- **Bacon**

- **Beef (high-fat cuts)**

- **Full-fat dairy** (e.g., butter, cheese, cream, ice cream)

- **High-fat foods** (especially those high in saturated fats or trans fats)

- **High-sodium foods**

- **Packaged and processed foods**

- **Packaged, processed meat alternatives**

- **Refined added sugars** (brown sugar, confectioners sugar, high fructose corn syrup, white sugar)

## Meal Prep

| Day | Breakfast | Lunch | Snack | Dinner |
|---|---|---|---|---|
| 1 | Ginger-Peach Oatmeal P - 14 | Salmon salad P - 23 | Shrimp and Grapefruit Salad P - 24 | Cabbage and Chickpea Salad P - 45 |
| 2 | Blueberry Walnut Yogurt Parfait P - 15 | Salmon curry recipe P - 25 | Salmon fish cakes P - 25 | Sweet Potato and Black BeanEnchilada P - 46 |
| 3 | Carrot Cake Oatmeal P - 19 | Shrimp with Quinoa P - 26 | Tuna Steaks with Mango Salsa P - 26 | Cashew Alfredo Pasta P - 51 |
| 4 | Avocado and Chickpea Sandwich P - 37 | Pistachio Salmon P - 27 | Tuna Stuffed Avocado Recipe P - 27 | Chicken Hash Recipe P - 54 |
| 5 | Ginger-Peach Oatmeal P - 14 | Salmon with Carrots and Broccoli P - 34 | Teriyaki Salmon with Mango P - 30 | Mango and Grilled Chicken Salad P - 56 |
| 6 | Pumpkin Spice Oatmeal P - 18 | Feta, and olive salad P - 37 | Fiery Prawns P - 31 | Chayote Chicken Noodle Soup P - 56 |
| 7 | Vegan Black Bean Burgers P - 38 | Vegan Black Bean Burgers P - 38 | Coconut Chicken Tenders P - 54 | Zucchini Noodle Pad Thai P - 47 |
| 8 | Almond Butter Banana Pancakes P - 14 | Avocado and White Bean Salad P - 43 | Green Tea Chia Pudding P - 62 | Mushroom & Spinach Quinoa Pilaf P - 46 |
| 9 | Blueberry Walnut Yogurt Parfait P - 15 | Tilapia with Broccoli P - 29 | Chia Seed and Blueberry Pudding P - 63 | Grilled Chicken and Quinoa Salad p - 60 |

| Day | Breakfast | Lunch | Snack | Dinner |
|---|---|---|---|---|
| 10 | Berry Almond Overnight Oats P - 16 | Avocado and Chickpea Sandwich P - 37 | Jamaican Chicken Fajitas P - 58 | Seafood Paella P - 30 |
| 11 | Pumpkin Seed and Oat Breakfast Bars P - 22 | Prawn and Broccoli Coconut Curry P - 28 | Carrot Cake Bites P - 66 | Zucchini Noodle with Almond Butter P - 51 |
| 12 | Quinoa & Berry Breakfast Bowl P - 17 | Tuna Steaks with Mango Salsa P - 26 | Coconut soup with shrimp P - 32 | Easy coconut chicken P - 55 |
| 13 | Anti-Inflammatory Bowl P - 22 | Chickpea and Avocado Wrap P - 41 | Tuna Poke Bowl Recipe P - 33 | Roasted chicken thighs P - 52 |
| 14 | Avocado Deviled Eggs P - 15 | Roasted Cauliflower Salad P - 42 | Blueberry and Lemon Muffins P - 65 | Pomegranate Chicken Salad P - 57 |
| 15 | Pumpkin Spice Oatmeal p - 18 | Roasted Veggie and Farro Bowl P - 42 | Teriyaki Salmon with Mango P - 30 | Sweet Potato and Kale Tacos P - 47 |
| 16 | Tofu Scramble with Spinach P - 20 | Cauliflower Tacos P - 38 | Tuna Stuffed Avocado Recipe P - 27 | Marinated Grilled Chicken P - 57 |
| 17 | Turmeric Oats Bowl P - 21 | Protein-Packed Tofu Scramble P - 41 | Blueberry and Lemon Muffins P - 65 | Herbed Turkey and Vegetable Soup P - 58 |
| 18 | Cucumber Avocado Toast P - 17 | Mediterranean Quinoa Salad P - 39 | Carrot Cake Bites P - 66 | Easy Chicken + Spinach P - 55 |

| Day | Breakfast | Lunch | Snack | Dinner |
|---|---|---|---|---|
| 19 | Avocado Deviled Eggs P - 15 | Lemon Basil Salmon P - 29 | Fiery Prawns P - 31 | Vegan Spaghetti Carbonara P - 50 |
| 20 | Cucumber Avocado Toast p - 17 | Tuna and White Bean Salad P - 35 | Green Tea Chia Pudding P - 62 | Asian Cabbage and edamame Salad P - 44 |
| 21 | Pear & Walnut Oatmeal p - 18 | Creamy leek and salmon soup P - 32 | Cauliflower Rice & Black Bean Bowl P - 49 | Pumpkin and Spinach Curry P - 48 |
| 22 | Zucchini & Onion Frittata P - 16 | Walnut-Crusted Salmon P - 36 | Tuna and Strawberry Salad P - 33 | Asian Soup with Chicken Meatballs P - 53 |
| 23 | Ginger Pear Breakfast Salad P - 20 | Vegan Shepherd's Pie P - 40 | Coconut Chicken Tenders P - 54 | Mushroom Risotto P - 50 |
| 24 | Quinoa & Berry Breakfast Bowl p - 17 | Salmon and Avocado Toast P - 36 | Cajun Jumbo Shrimp P - 34 | Chicken bulgogi P - 53 |
| 25 | Pear & Walnut Oatmeal P - 18 | Butternut Squash Risotto P - 40 | Chia Seed and Blueberry Pudding P - 63 | Creamy Spinach & Artichoke Pasta P - 48 |
| 26 | Berry Almond Overnight Oats P - 16 | Mushroom Stroganoff P - 39 | Salmon fish cakes P - 25 | Moroccan Chickpea Soup P - 49 |
| 27 | Scallion Pancake P - 21 | Pan-Seared Tuna Steaks P - 35 | Salmon Niçoise Salad P - 24 | Turkey Patties P - 52 |

| Day | Breakfast | Lunch | Snack | Dinner |
|---|---|---|---|---|
| 28 | Zucchini & Onion Frittata<br>P - 16 | Salmon with fennel salad<br>P - 31 | Cajun Jumbo Shrimp<br>P - 34 | Lentil & Carrot Salad<br>P - 44 |
| 29 | Coconut Milk Chia Pudding<br>P - 19 | Cod and Asparagus<br>P - 28 | Cauliflower Rice & Black Bean Bowl<br>P - 49 | Sprouts and Walnut Salad<br>P - 45 |
| 30 | Almond Butter Banana Pancakes<br>P - 14 | Shrimp fried rice<br>P - 23 | Tuna Poke Bowl Recipe<br>p - 33 | Sweet Potato & Black Bean Bowl<br>P - 43 |

# Breakfast

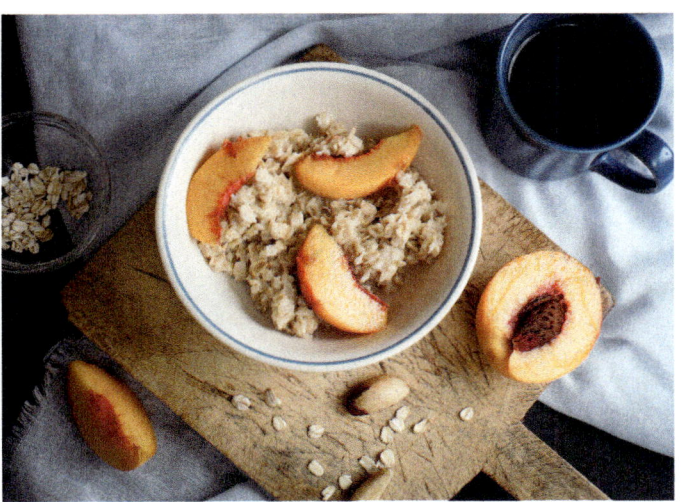

## Ginger-Peach Oatmeal

### Ingredients

- 1/2 cup rolled oats
- 1 cup water
- 1 sliced peach
- 1/2 tsp grated ginger
- a drizzle of honey

### Instructions

Cook oats with water and grated ginger. Once cooked, top with fresh peach slices and a drizzle of honey.

**Servings-1, Calories: 250**
**Proteins: 6, Fats: 3, Carbs: 52**

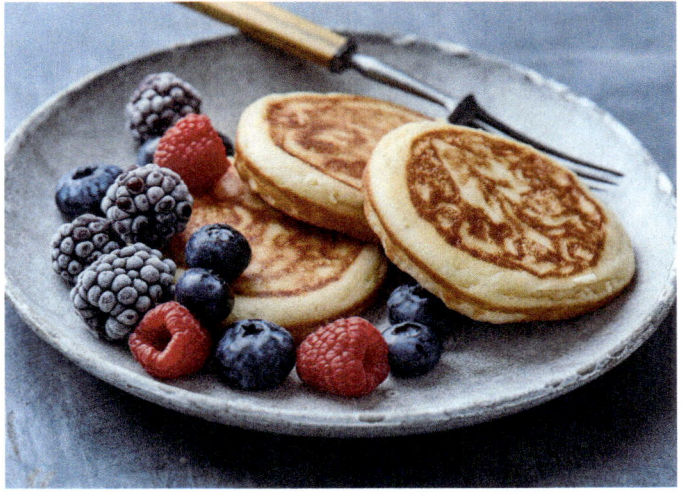

## Almond Butter Banana Pancakes

### Ingredients

- 1 ripe banana
- 2 eggs
- 1/4 cup almond flour
- 1 tbsp almond butter
- 1/2 tsp baking powder

### Instructions

Mix the banana with eggs, almond flour, almond butter, and baking powder. Cook spoonful's on a hot pan until bubbles form, then flip and cook the other side.

**Servings-2, Calories: 270**
**Proteins: 10, Fats: 18, Carbs: 20**

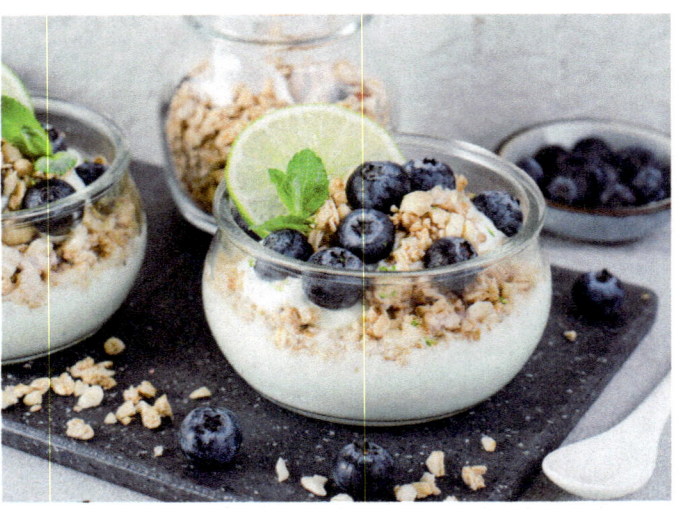

## Blueberry Walnut Yogurt Parfait

### Ingredients

- 3/4 cup Greek yogurt
- 1/2 cup blueberries
- 1/4 cup walnuts
- Sprinkle of cinnamon

### Instructions

Layer Greek yogurt with blueberries and walnuts in a glass. Sprinkle with cinnamon.

**Servings-1, Calories: 320**
**Proteins: 15, Fats: 21, Carbs: 23**

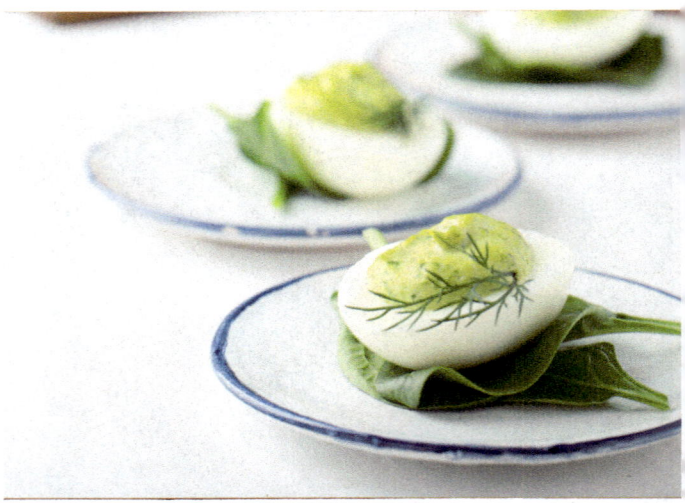

## Avocado Deviled Eggs

### Ingredients

- 5-7 eggs
- Chilli (1/4 teaspoon)
- 1 avocado
- Paprika (1/4 teaspoon)
- Salt (1/4 teaspoon)
- Cumin (1/4 teaspoon)
- Garlic (1/4 teaspoon)
- Cilantro (2 tablespoon)
- Pepper (1/4 teaspoon)

### Instructions

Boil the eggs in a pot of water for 15-20 minutes. Let them cool, then remove the shells. Cut the eggs lengthwise and remove the yolks. Mix the yolks with the spices until combined. Fill the egg halves with the mixture and top with lime juice and cilantro.

**Servings-7, Kcal- 91**
**Proteins- 8g, Fats- 15g, Carbs- 1g**

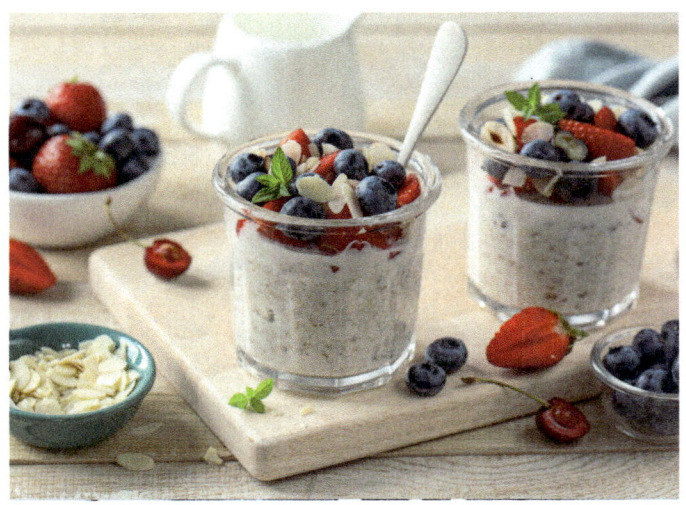

## Berry Almond Overnight Oats

### Ingredients

- 1/2 cup mixed berries (blueberries, raspberries, strawberries)
- 1/2 cup rolled oats
- 1/2 cup almond milk
- 1 tablespoon chia seeds
- 1 tablespoon sliced almonds
- 1/2 teaspoon vanilla extract
- 1 tablespoon honey

### Instructions

Combine rolled oats, almond milk, chia seeds, and vanilla extract in a jar. Mix well—top with mixed berries and sliced almonds. Seal the jar and refrigerate overnight. In the morning, stir the oats, add honey if desired, and enjoy cold.

**Servings-1, Kcal- 350**
**Proteins- 10g, Fats- 10g, Carbs- 50g**

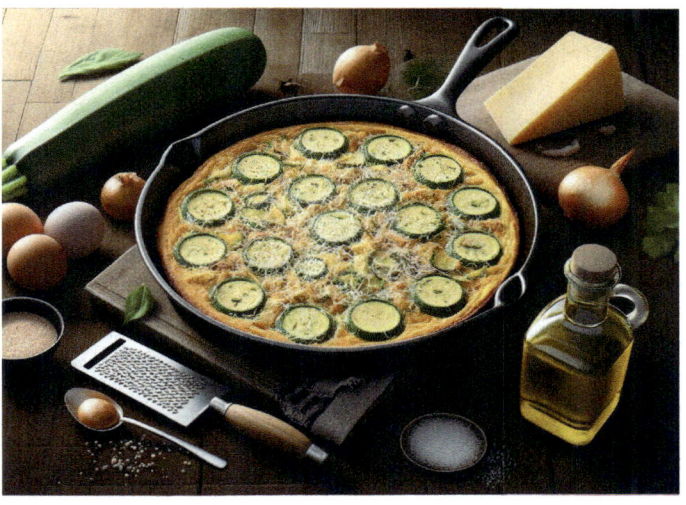

## Zucchini & Onion Frittata

### Ingredients

- 4 eggs
- 1 zucchini, sliced
- 1/2 onion, diced
- 1 tablespoon olive oil
- Salt and pepper to taste
- 1/4 cup grated Parmesan

### Instructions

Sauté zucchini and onion in olive oil until soft. Beat eggs and pour over the vegetables, cooking until the eggs are set. Sprinkle Parmesan cheese on top and broil until golden.

**Servings-1, Kcal- 350**
**Proteins- 22g, Fats- 25g, Carbs- 8**

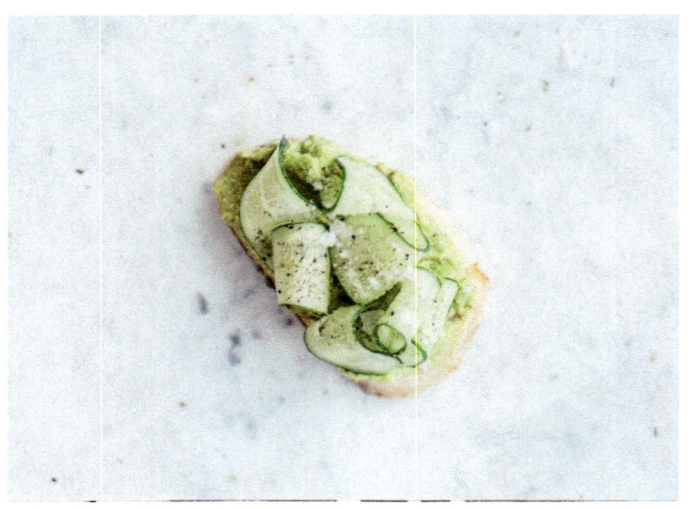

## Cucumber Avocado Toast

### Ingredients

- 1 slice whole-grain bread, toasted
- 1/2 avocado, mashed
- 1/4 cucumber, sliced
- Lemon juice
- Salt and pepper to taste

### Instructions

Spread mashed avocado on toasted bread—top with cucumber slices, a squeeze of lemon juice, and season with salt and pepper.

**Servings-1, Kcal- 250**
**Proteins- 6g, Fats- 15g, Carbs- 20**

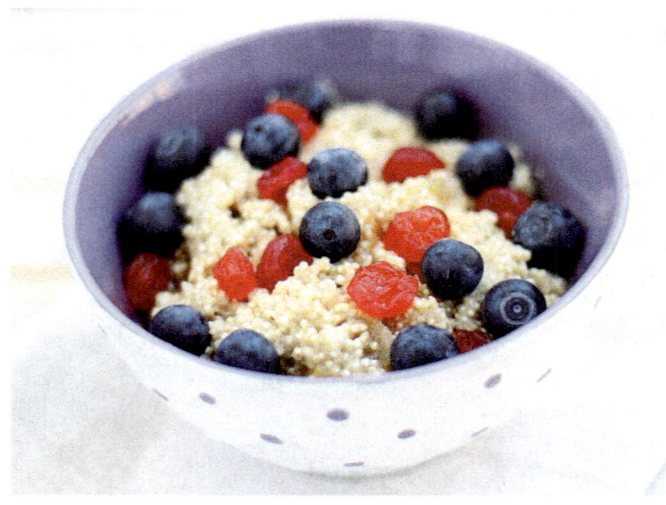

## Quinoa & Berry Breakfast Bowl

### Ingredients

- 1/2 cup cooked quinoa
- 1/2 cup mixed berries
- 1 tablespoon walnuts, chopped
- 1 teaspoon cinnamon
- A drizzle of maple syrup (optional)

### Instructions

Mix cooked quinoa with cinnamon and walnuts. Top with mixed berries and a drizzle of maple syrup if desired.

**Servings-1, Kcal- 300**
**Proteins- 8g, Fats- 8g, Carbs- 45**

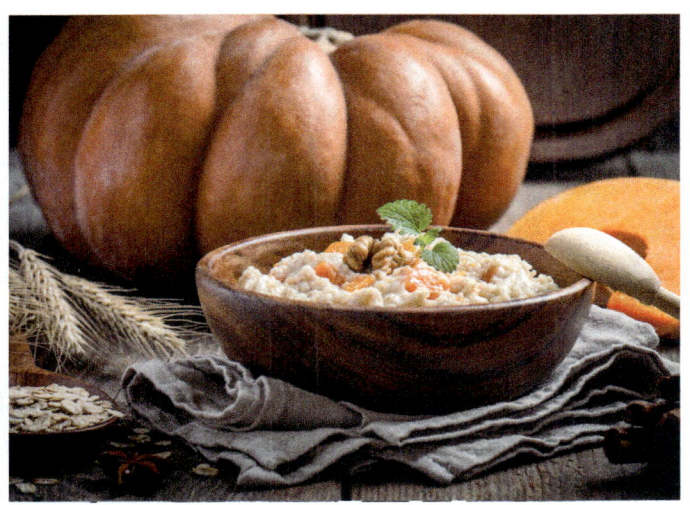

## Pumpkin Spice Oatmeal

### Ingredients

- 1/2 cup rolled oats
- 1 cup almond milk
- 1/4 cup pumpkin puree
- 1/2 tsp pumpkin pie spice
- 1 tablespoon pumpkin seeds
- A drizzle of honey

### Instructions

Cook oats in almond milk, stirring in pumpkin puree and pumpkin pie spice. Serve topped with pumpkin seeds and honey if desired.

**Servings-1, Kcal- 280**
**Proteins- 10g, Fats- 6g, Carbs- 50**

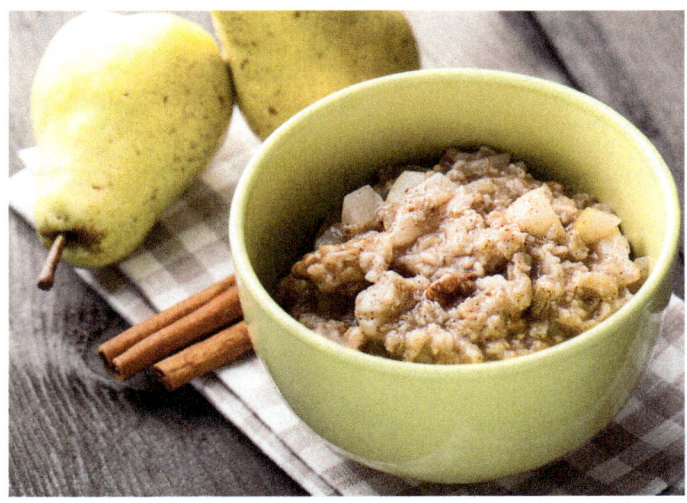

## Pear & Walnut Oatmeal

### Ingredients

- 1/2 cup rolled oats
- 1 cup water or almond milk
- 1 pear, diced
- 1 tbsp walnuts, chopped
- 1/2 teaspoon cinnamon

### Instructions

Cook oats with water or almond milk, stir in cinnamon. Top with pear and walnuts before serving.

**Servings-1, Kcal- 300**
**Proteins- 8g, Fats- 10g, Carbs- 45**

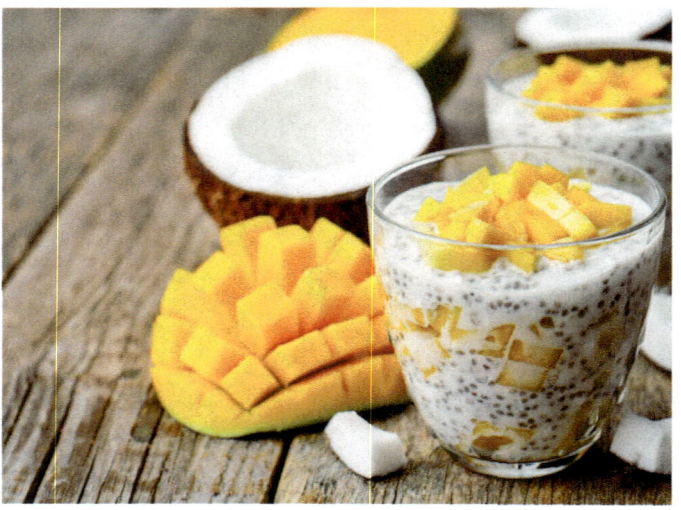

## Coconut Milk Chia Pudding

### Ingredients

- 1/4 cup chia seeds
- 1 cup coconut milk
- 1/2 teaspoon vanilla extract
- 1 tbsp shredded coconut
- 1/2 cup mango, diced

### Instructions

Mix chia seeds with coconut milk and vanilla, and let sit until thickened. Top with shredded coconut and mango before serving.

**Servings-1, Kcal- 350**
**Proteins- 8g, Fats- 20g, Carbs- 30**

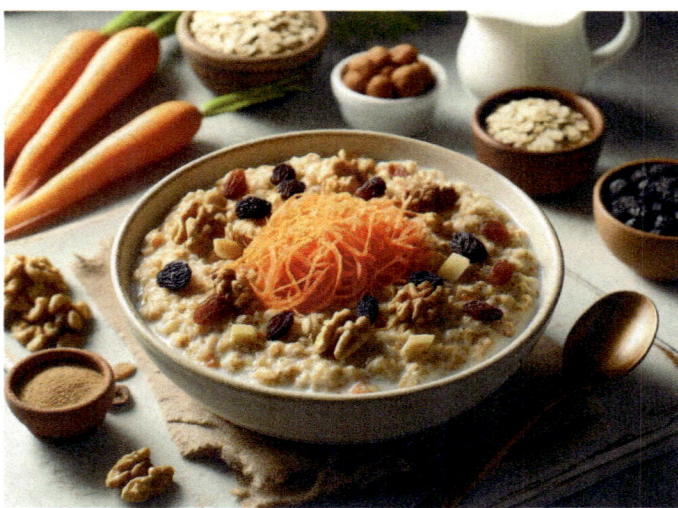

## Carrot Cake Oatmeal

### Ingredients

- 1/2 cup rolled oats
- 1 cup almond milk
- 1/2 cup grated carrots
- 1/2 teaspoon cinnamon
- 1/4 teaspoon nutmeg
- 1 tbsp chopped walnuts
- 1 tablespoon raisins
- Drizzle of maple syrup

### Instructions

Cook oats in almond milk with grated carrots, cinnamon, and nutmeg. Stir in walnuts and raisins. Serve with a drizzle of maple syrup if desired.

**Servings-1, Kcal- 320**
**Proteins- 8g, Fats- 8g, Carbs- 55**

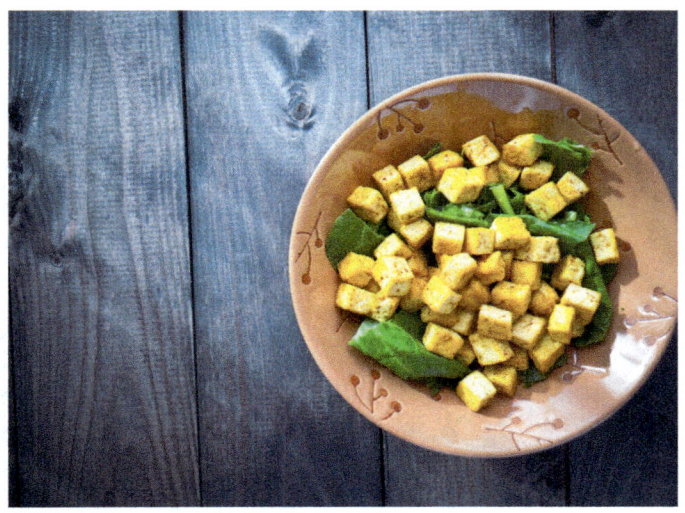

## Tofu Scramble with Spinach

### Ingredients

- 1/2 block firm tofu, crumbled
- 1 cup spinach leaves
- 1/4 onion, diced
- Salt and pepper to taste
- 1 tablespoon olive oil
- 1/2 teaspoon turmeric

### Instructions

Sauté onion in olive oil until softened. Add crumbled tofu and turmeric, and cook for a few minutes. Stir in spinach until wilted; season with salt and pepper.

**Servings-1, Kcal- 250**
**Proteins- 14g, Fats- 18g, Carbs- 10**

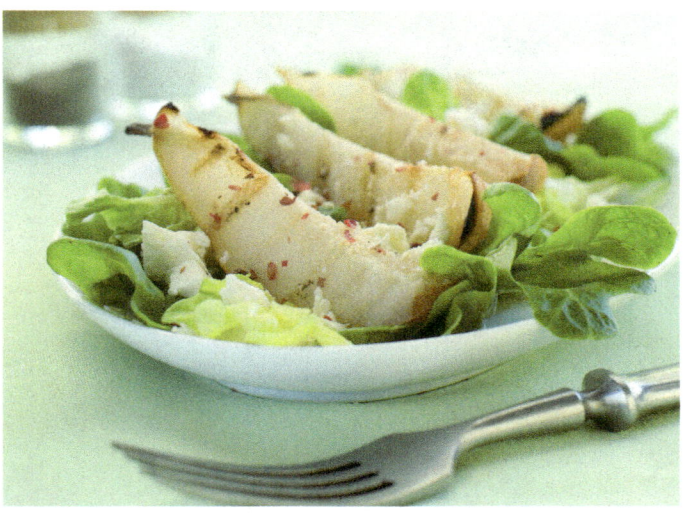

## Ginger Pear Breakfast Salad

### Ingredients

- 2 cups mixed greens
- 1 pear, sliced
- 1 tbsp chopped walnuts
- 1/4 tsp grated ginger
- 1 tablespoon balsamic vinegar

### Instructions

Toss mixed greens with pear slices and walnuts. Mix grated ginger with balsamic vinegar and drizzle over the salad.

**Servings-1, Kcal- 150**
**Proteins- 3g, Fats- 7g, Carbs- 20**

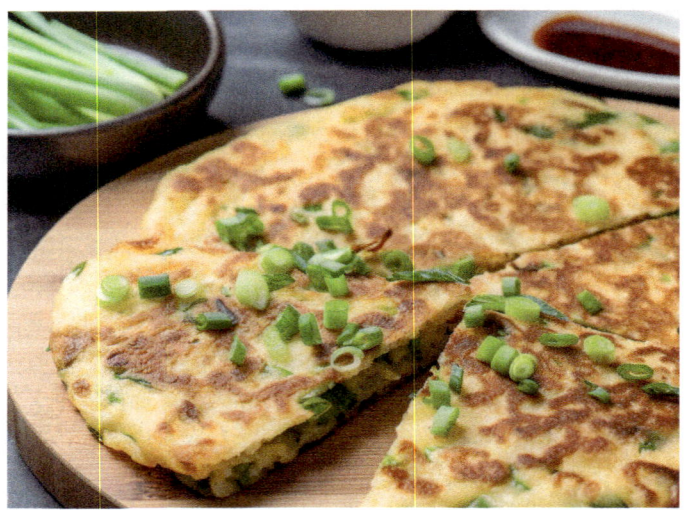

## Scallion Pancake

### Ingredients

- 1 cup all-purpose flour
- 1/3 cup hot water
- 2 tablespoons sesame oil
- 2 scallions, finely chopped
- 1/4 teaspoon salt
- 2 tablespoons vegetable oil

### Instructions

Mix flour with hot water to form a dough and let it rest for 20 minutes. Roll it out thinly, brush with sesame oil, sprinkle with salt, and add scallions. Roll it into a log, coil it, and flatten it. Fry in vegetable oil for 2-3 minutes per side until golden. Slice and serve hot.

**Servings-2, Calories: 230**
**Carbs: 25 g, Fat: 12 g, Protein: 5 g**

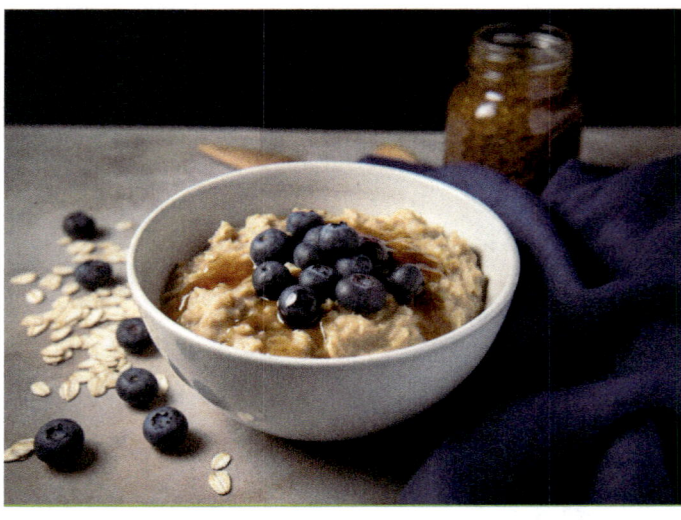

## Turmeric Oats Bowl

### Ingredients

- 1/2 cup rolled oats
- 1 cup almond milk
- 1/2 tsp turmeric powder
- Pinch of black pepper
- 1 tbsp honey
- 1/4 cup blue berries
- 1 tbsp chopped almonds

### Instructions

Cook the oats with almond milk, turmeric, and black pepper on the stove according to the oats package directions. Once cooked, stir in the honey and top with blueberries and chopped almonds.

**Servings-1, Calories: 339**
**Carbs: 60 g, Fat: 9 g, Protein: 8 g**

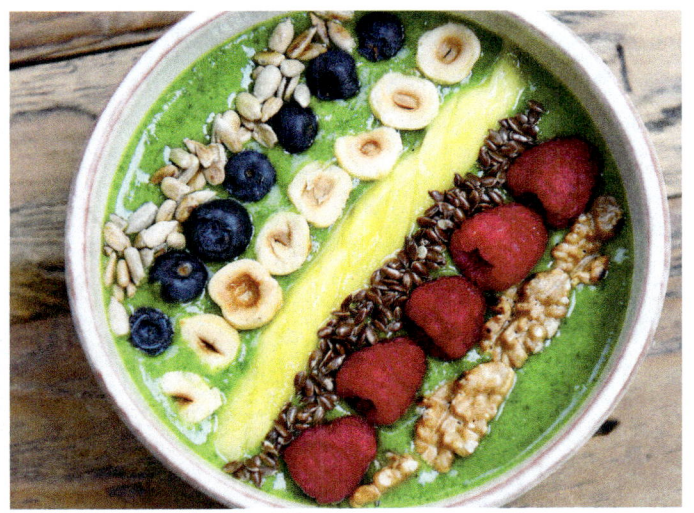

## Anti-Inflammatory Bowl

### Ingredients

- 1 cup spinach
- 1/2 cup mango chunks
- 1/2 banana
- 1/4 avocado
- 1 tablespoon ground flaxseed
- 1 cup coconut water

### Instructions

Blend all ingredients until smooth. Pour into a bowl and add toppings of your choice (e.g., sliced walnuts, seeds, fresh berries).

**Servings-1, Calories: 320**
**Carbs: 51 g, Fat: 10 g, Protein: 5 g**

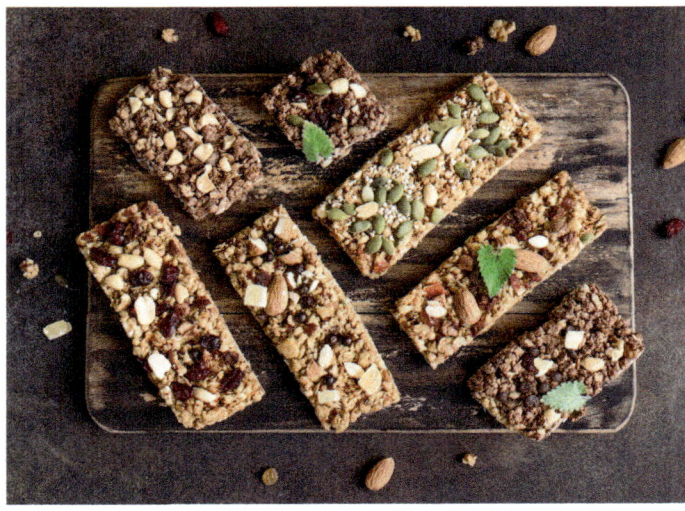

## Pumpkin Seed and Oat Breakfast Bars

### Ingredients

- 1 cup rolled oats
- 1/2 cup pumpkin seeds
- 1/4 cup honey
- 1/4 cup applesauce
- 1/2 teaspoon cinnamon
- 1/4 teaspoon salt
- 1/2 cup dried cherries or cranberries

### Instructions

Preheat oven to 350°F (175°C), lining a dish with parchment. Combine oats, pumpkin seeds, cinnamon, and salt; mix in honey and applesauce. Add cherries or cranberries. Press into the dish and bake for 20-25 minutes until golden. Cool before slicing into bars. For Air fyer: Air fry at 175°C (350°F) for 15-18 minutes until golden.

**Serving: 1, Calories: 150**
**Proteins: 4, Fats: 5, Carbs: 22**

# SEA FOOD

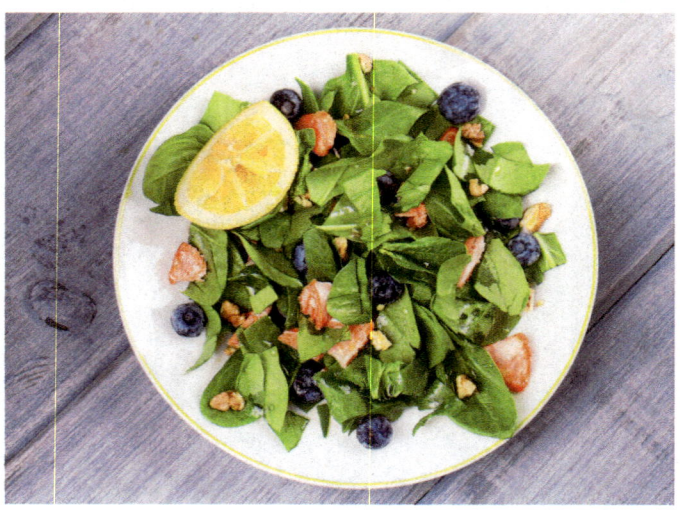

## Salmon salad

### Ingredients

- Fresh spinach: 4 cups (about 120g)
- Cooked salmon (flaked or cut into small pieces): 1 cup (about 200g)
- Walnuts: 1/2 cup (about 60g), roughly chopped
- Fresh blueberries: 1 cup (about 150g)
- Optional dressing: 2 tablespoons olive oil, 1 tablespoon balsamic vinegar, and a pinch of salt and pepper.

### Instructions

Mix spinach, walnuts, blueberries, and cooked salmon pieces in a large bowl. Drizzle with the dressing, or enjoy it plain for a lighter option.

**Servings-2, Kcal- 550**
**Proteins- 26g, Fats- 45g, Carbs- 18g**

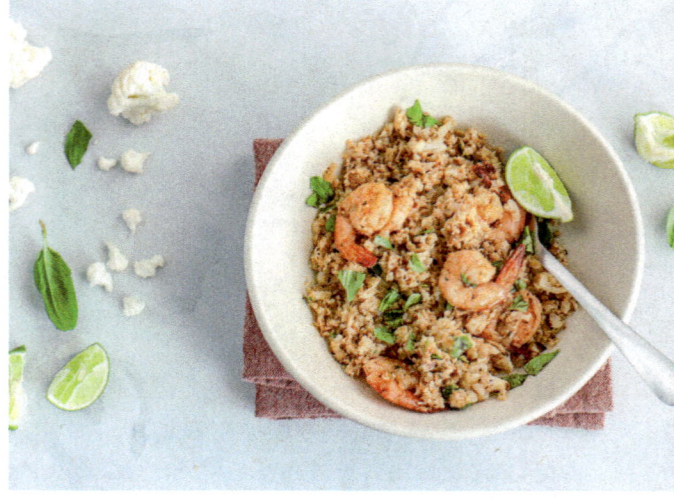

## Shrimp fried rice

### Ingredients

- 1 tablespoon sesame oil
- 3 green onions
- ½ tablespoon soy sauce
- 2 tablespoons of coconut oil
- 2 eggs (beaten)
- 1 ½ cup cauliflower rice
- ½ pound shrimp (250 gram)

### Instructions

In a pan heat 1 tablespoon of coconut oil, add shrimp, and cook for 3-5 minutes. Remove from pan and set aside. Heat another tablespoon of coconut oil, add onions, and cauliflower rice. Cook for 6 minutes approx. Add soy sauce and eggs to the pan and stir continuously. Add sesame oil and stir, then toss with shrimp and serve.

**Servings-2, Kcal- 505**
**Proteins- 42g, Fats- 34g, Carbs- 3g**

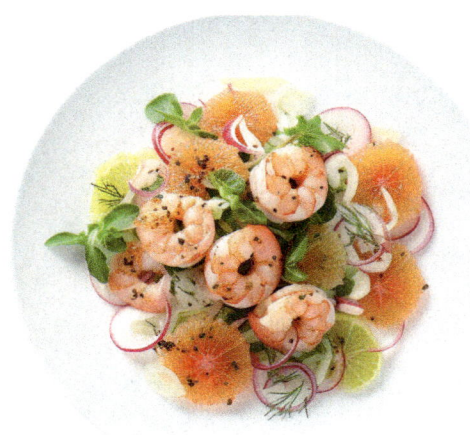
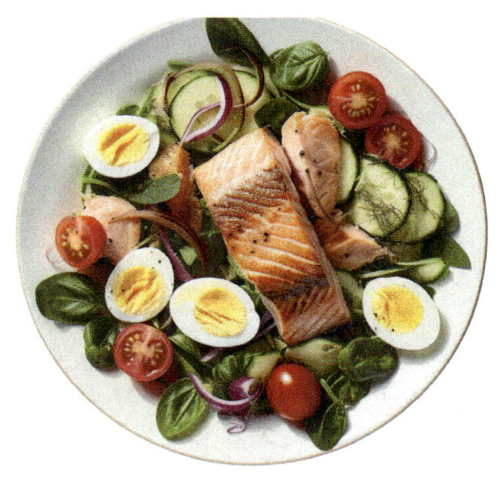

## Shrimp and Grapefruit Salad

### Ingredients

- Crushed red pepper flakes (1/4 tsp)
- Olive oil (2 tablespoons)
- Cucumber, thinly sliced (1 medium)
- Shrimp, peeled and deveined (1 lb.)
- Sea salt and black pepper, to taste
- Red onion, thinly sliced (1 small)
- Fennel seeds (1/4 teaspoon)
- Mixed salad greens (4 cups)
- Grapefruit, sliced (2 large)
- Olive oil (2 tablespoons)
- Avocado, sliced (1 ripe)
- Lime, juice of (1 lime)
- Honey (1 tablespoon)

### Instructions

Sauté seasoned shrimp in oil for 2-3 minutes, then cool. Toss greens, onion, avocado, cucumber, and grapefruit. Whisk olive oil, lime juice, honey, spices, salt, and pepper for dressing. Arrange salad, top with shrimp, drizzle dressing.

**Servings-3, Kcal- 660**
**Proteins- 57g, Fats- 27g, Carbs- 40g**

## Salmon Niçoise Salad

### Ingredients

- Lemon, juice of (1 lemon)
- Black olives, pitted (1/2 cup)
- Mixed salad greens (4 cups)
- Dijon mustard (1 tablespoon)
- Cherry tomatoes, halved (1 cup)
- Hard-boiled eggs, quartered (4)
- Sea salt and black pepper (to taste)
- Fresh parsley, chopped (for garnish)
- Salmon fillets (4 fillets / 6 ounces each )
- Green beans, trimmed (1 cup)
- Olive oil (3 tablespoons, extra for grill)
- Small baby potatoes, boiled (1 lb.)

### Instructions

Grill seasoned salmon for 3-4 minutes per side. Toss green beans, potatoes, tomatoes, olives, and eggs. Whisk olive oil, lemon juice, Dijon, salt, and pepper. Arrange greens, top with salmon, drizzle dressing, garnish with parsley, and serve!

**Servings-4, Kcal- 582**
**Proteins- 47g, Fats- 33g, Carbs- 29g**

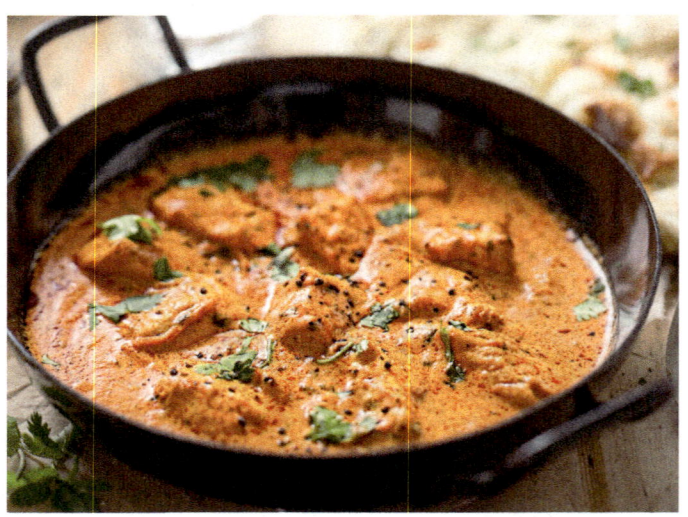

## Salmon curry recipe

### Ingredients

- 1/2 medium onion, diced
- 2 cups of broth
- 2 cups of green beans, diced
- 450 g raw salmon, diced
- 1.5 tablespoons of curry powder
- 2 tablespoons of coconut oil
- 1 teaspoon garlic powder
- Salt and pepper
- Cream from coconut milk
- 2 tablespoons of basil

### Instructions

Fry diced onion in coconut oil until translucent. Add green beans and fry for few more minutes. Add broth or water and bring to a boil. Add curry powder, garlic, and salmon. Add coconut cream and simmer until the salmon is cooked (3-5 minutes). Garnish with salt, pepper, and chopped basil.

**Servings-3, Kcal- 400**
**Proteins- 50g, Fats- 23g, Carbs- 3g**

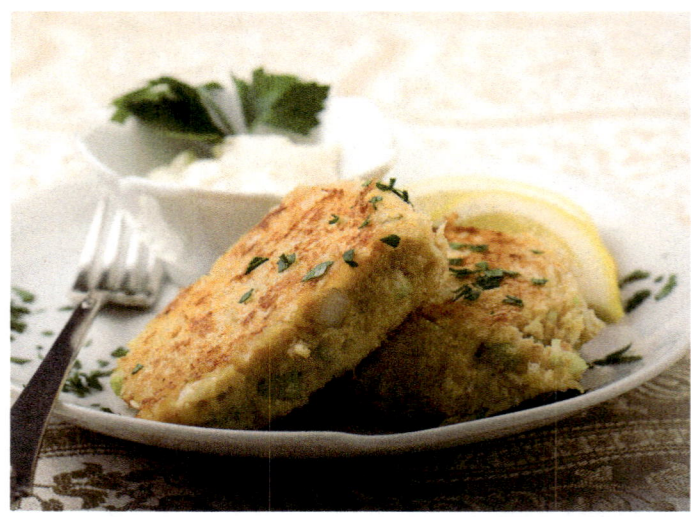

## Salmon fish cakes

### Ingredients

- 3 cans of salmon
- 1/4 cup of coconut oil (60 ml)
- 2 tablespoons of fresh dill
- Salt and pepper, to taste
- 3 medium eggs, whisked
- 1/4 cup shredded coconut (20 g)
- 1/4 cup of coconut flour
- 2 tablespoons of coconut oil

### Instructions

Combine the ingredients for the fish cake in a large bowl. Form the mixture into 8 patties. Melt 2 tablespoons (30 ml) of coconut oil in a large pan. Carefully place the patties in the oil. Cook until golden brown on both sides for about 3 to 4 minutes.

**Servings-8, Kcal- 177**
**Proteins- 20g, Fats- 8g, Carbs- 3g**

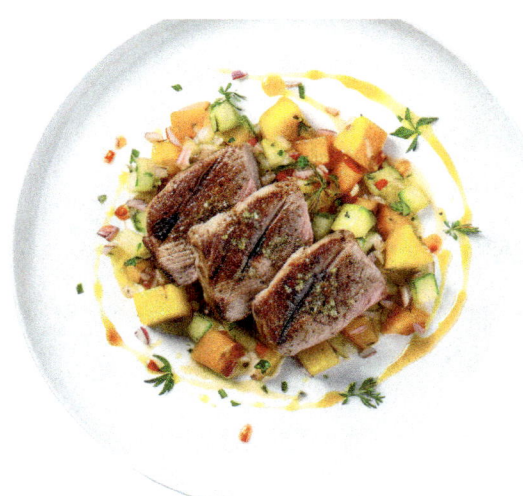
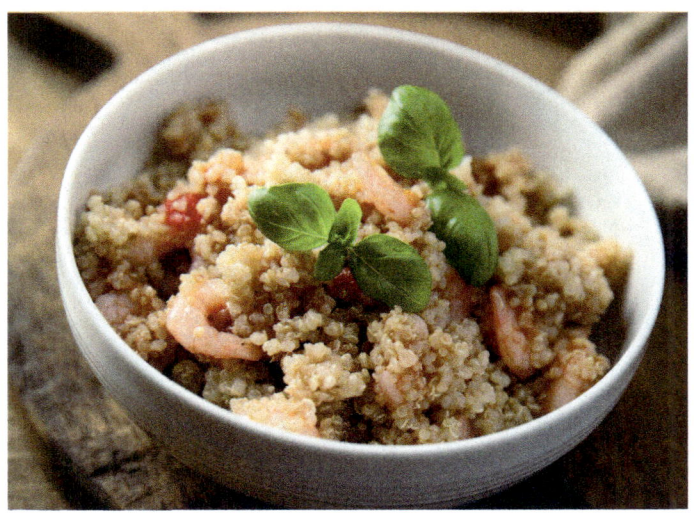

## Tuna Steaks with Mango Salsa

### Ingredients

**Tuna Steaks:** Olive oil (3 tablespoons)
- Garlic cloves, minced (2)
- Tuna steaks (3-4 pieces/ 6-8 oz)
- Sea salt and black pepper, to taste
- Fresh lime, zest and juice of (1 lime)
- Fresh cilantro, chopped (2 tbsp)

**Mango Salsa:** Sea salt, to taste
- Fresh lime, juice of (1)
- Jalapeño, diced (1, optional)
- Red onion, Cilantro (1/4 cup)
- Mango, peeled and diced (1 large)

### Instructions

Whisk oil, lime zest, juice, garlic, salt, pepper, and cilantro. Marinate tuna for 15-30 minutes. Grill for 2-3 minutes per side. Mix mango, onion, cilantro, lime juice, and jalapeño for salsa. Serve tuna with salsa on top.

**Servings-4, Kcal- 240**
**Proteins- 37g, Fats- 8g, Carbs- 16g**

## Shrimp with Quinoa

### Ingredients

- 1 lb shrimp, peeled and deveined
- 1 tbsp olive oil
- 1/2 tsp chili powder
- 1/2 tsp paprika
- 1 cup quinoa, cooked
- Salt and pepper to taste
- Lemon wedges for serving

### Instructions

Preheat grill to medium-high. Toss shrimp with olive oil, chili powder, paprika, salt, and pepper—grill shrimp until opaque, about 2 minutes per side. Serve over cooked quinoa with lemon wedges.

**Serving: 1, Calories: 380**
**Proteins: 35, Fats: 10, Carbs: 35**

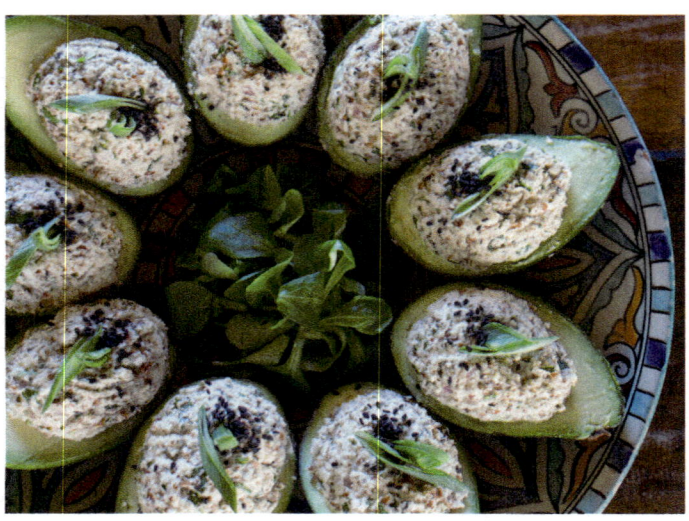

## Tuna Stuffed Avocado Recipe

### Ingredients

- 1 (5 oz.) can tuna
- Pinch of dried dill
- 2 tablespoons greek yogurt
- Salt and pepper
- 1 medium avocado (cut in half and pit removed)

### Instructions

Combine tuna, Greek yogurt and dill in a small mixing bowl. Season it with salt and pepper as desired. Fill the avocado halves with tuna salad and serve.

**Servings-1, Kcal- 340**
**Proteins- 20g, Fats- 25g, Carbs- 3g**

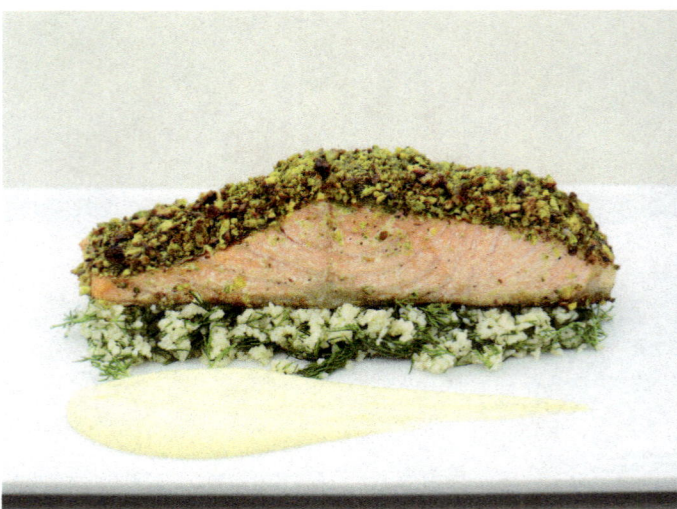

## Pistachio Salmon

### Ingredients

- 1/3 cup pistachios, finely chopped
- 1 salmon fillet (1 pound)
- 2 tablespoons of panko bread crumb
- 1/2 teaspoon salt
- 1/4 cup grated Parmesan cheese
- 1/4 teaspoon pepper

### Instructions

Preheat the oven to 200 ° C. Combine the pistachios with breadcrumbs and cheese in a flat bowl. Place salmon on 15 x 10 x 1 inch greased aluminum foil. Skin side down; sprinkle with salt and pepper. Garnish with the pistachio mixture. Bake uncovered until the fish peels off easily with a fork, 15 to 20 minutes. For Air Fryer: Air fry at 200°C (400°F) for 10-12 minutes until the salmon flakes easily with a fork.

**Servings-2, Kcal- 515**
**Proteins- 80g, Fats- 17g, Carbs- 4g**

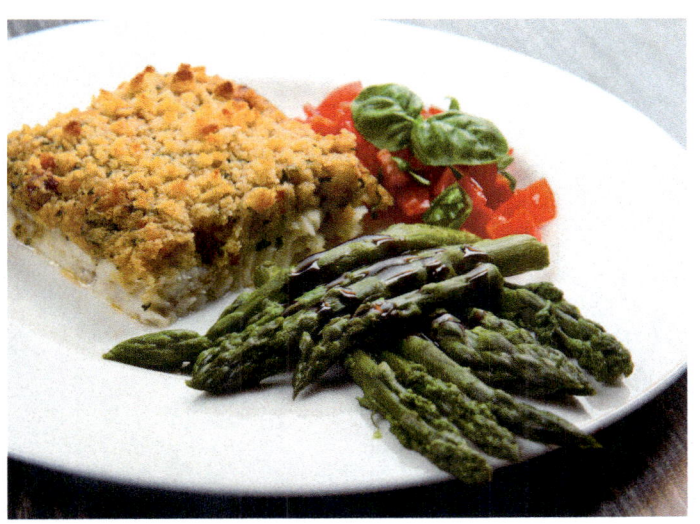

## Cod and Asparagus

### Ingredients

- 4 cod fillets (4 ounces each )
- 2 tablespoons of lemon juice
- 1&1/2 teaspoons of grated lemon zest
- 1 pound asparagus, trimmed
- 1/4 cup grated Romano cheese

### Instructions

Preheat the oven to 170 C. Add cod and asparagus to a baking pan. Brush the baking pan with oil. Brush the fish with lemon juice. Sprinkle with lemon zest. Sprinkle fish and vegetables with Romano cheese. Cook for about 12 minutes until the fish peels off easily with a fork. Take the pan out of the oven. Preheat broiler. Broil cod mixture 3-4 inches from the heat until the vegetables are lightly browned, 2-3 minutes. For Air Fryer: Air fry at 170°C (340°F) for 10-12 minutes, then broil at 200°C (400°F) for 2-3 minutes.

**Servings-4, Kcal- 312**
**Proteins- 60g, Fats- 9g, Carbs- 3g**

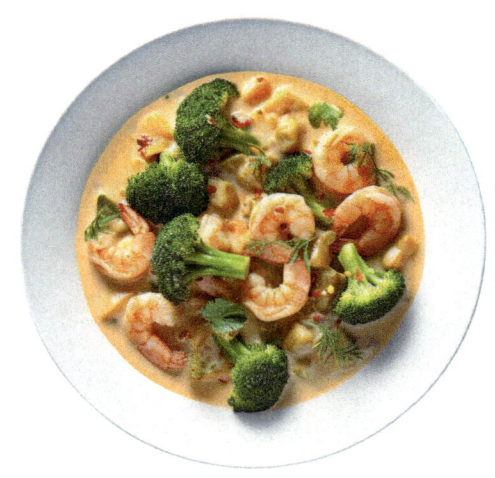

## Prawn and Broccoli Coconut Curry

### Ingredients

- Red chili flakes (1/4 teaspoon)
- Olive oil or coconut oil (2 tbsp)
- Prawns, peeled and deveined (1 lb.)
- Fresh ginger, grated (1 tablespoon)
- Sea salt and black pepper, to taste
- Coriander powder (1/2 teaspoon)
- Fresh cilantro, chopped (garnish)
- Lemongrass stalk, Onion (1)
- Coconut milk (1 can/ 13.5 oz)
- Garlic cloves, minced (3)
- Broccoli florets (3 cups)
- Turmeric (1 teaspoon)
- Cumin (1/2 teaspoon)

### Instructions

Heat oil, sauté onion for 2-3 minutes, then add garlic and ginger. Stir in spices, cook for a minute. Add lemongrass-infused coconut milk, bring to a simmer. Cook broccoli for 5 minutes, then add prawns and cook until pink. Remove lemongrass, season, and serve!

**Servings-4, Kcal- 310**
**Proteins- 23g, Fats- 19g, Carbs- 11g**

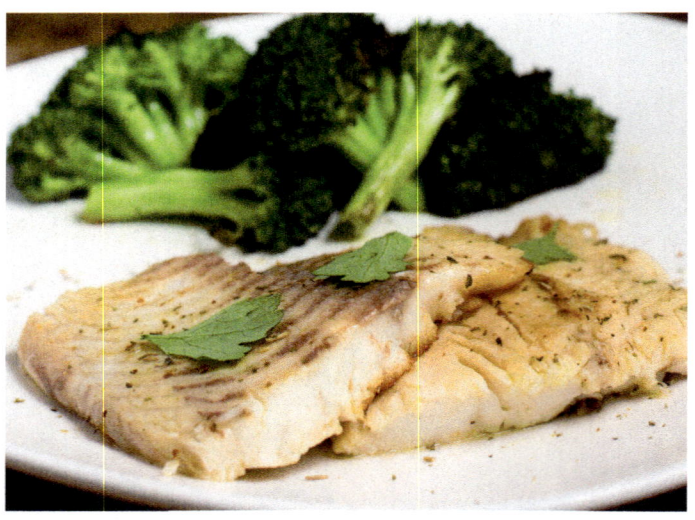

## Tilapia with Broccoli

### Ingredients

- Tilapia fillets: 4 (about 120g each)
- Broccoli florets: 4 cups (about 600g)
- Olive oil: 2 tablespoons
- Garlic: 2 cloves, minced
- Lemon juice: 2 tablespoons
- Salt and pepper: to taste
- Paprika: 1 teaspoon (optional for seasoning the fish)

### Instructions

Steam 4 cups of broccoli until tender-crisp and set aside. Heat 1 tbsp olive oil in a skillet, season 4 tilapia fillets with salt, pepper, and paprika, and cook for 3–4 minutes per side, squeezing lemon juice over them while cooking. Add olive oil, sauté minced garlic in the same skillet, and toss the broccoli for 2–3 minutes, seasoning with lemon juice, salt, and pepper. Serve the tilapia with the broccoli and garnish with lemon wedges.

**Servings-4, Kcal- 213**
**Proteins- 29g, Fats- 7g, Carbs- 11g**

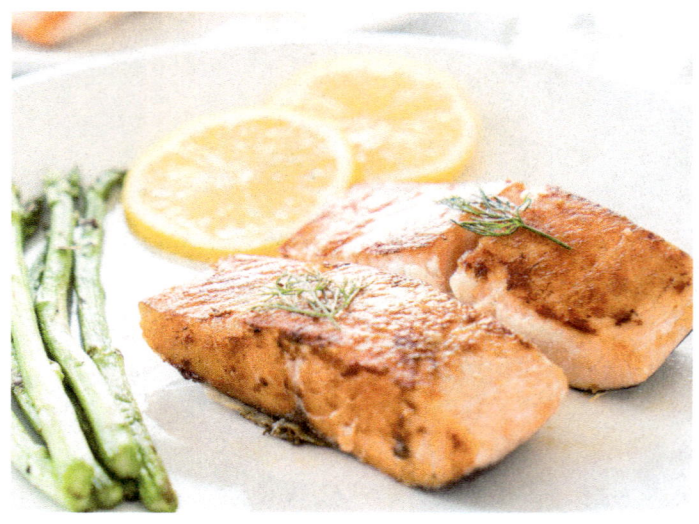

## Lemon Basil Salmon

### Ingredients

- 2 salmon fillets (5 ounces each)
- 1 tablespoon lemon juice
- 1 tablespoon olive oil
- 1/8 teaspoon pepper
- 1 tablespoon minced fresh basil
- 1/8 teaspoon salt
- Lemon wedges, optional

### Instructions

Place each fillet with the skin facing down on an aluminum foil. Combine oil, basil, lemon juice, salt, and pepper. Coat on the salmon. Fold the aluminum foil around the fish and close it tightly. Cook over a campfire or on a covered grill until the fish peels off easily with a fork (10-15 minutes). Open the aluminum foil carefully so that steam can escape. Serve with lemon wedges if desired. For Oven: Bake at 200°C (400°F) for 12-15 minutes

**Servings-2, Kcal- 200**
**Proteins- 39g, Fats- 5g, Carbs- 2g**

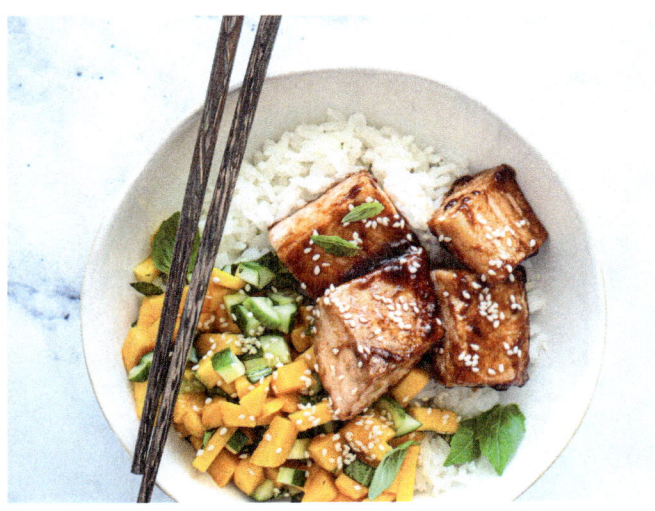

## Teriyaki Salmon with Mango

### Ingredients

- 2 salmon fillets (6 oz each)
- 2 tbsp coconut amino
- Honey, rice vinegar (1 tbsp )
- Grated ginger, Sesame oil (1 tsp )
- 1 garlic clove, minced
- 1 cup cooked jasmine rice
- Mango, cucumber (1/2)
- 1 tbsp sesame seeds
- 2 tbsp chopped green onions

### Instructions

Mix coconut amino, honey, rice vinegar, ginger, garlic, and sesame oil. Marinate salmon for 15 minutes. Heat a pan over medium heat, cook salmon for 3-4 minutes per side, basting with marinade until caramelized. Serve over cooked jasmine rice, topped with diced mango, cucumber, sesame seeds, and green onions.

**Servings-2, Calories: 475**
**Carbs: 50 g | Fat: 17 g | Protein: 33 g**

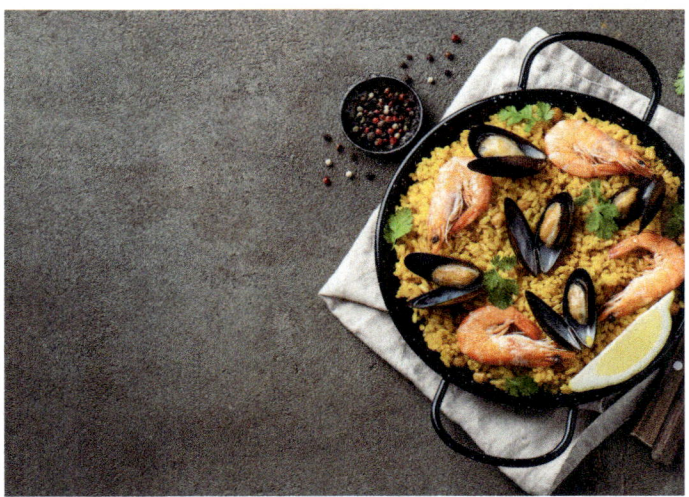

## Seafood Paella

### Ingredients

- 1 cup Arborio or short-grain rice
- 2 tbsp olive oil
- ½ onion, chopped
- 2 garlic cloves, minced
- Smoked paprika, Saffron threads (1/2 tsp)
- 1 small tomato, diced
- 2 ½ cups seafood broth
- Shrimp, Mussels (½ lb )
- ½ cup peas
- Salt and pepper to taste
- Lemon wedges and parsley for garnish

### Instructions

Heat olive oil, sauté onion, then add garlic, spices, and tomato. Stir in rice, broth, and simmer 15 minutes. Add seafood, cover, and cook 5-7 minutes. Stir in peas, season, and rest for 5 minutes. Garnish with parsley and lemon.

**Servings-4, Calories: 350**
**Proteins: 25, Fats: 10, Carbs: 45**

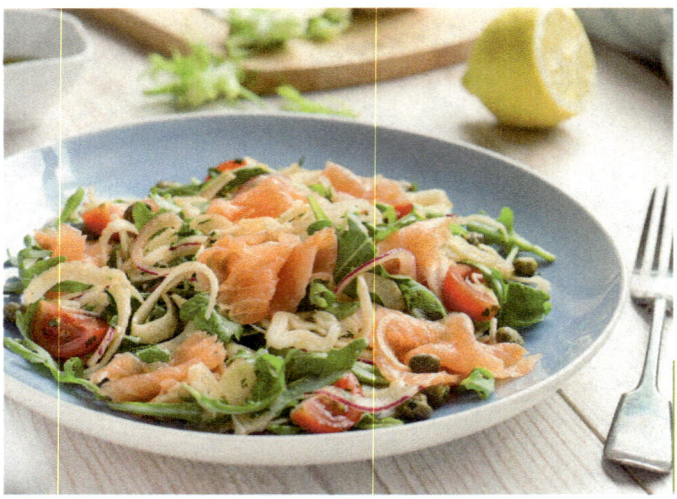

### Salmon with fennel salad

#### Ingredients

- 2 teaspoons of finely chopped parsley
- 1 teaspoon finely chopped thyme
- 1 teaspoon salt, split
- 4 salmon fillets cut in the middle
- 2 tablespoons olive oil
- 4 cups chopped fennel
- 2/3 cup of coconut yogurt
- 1 crushed garlic clove
- 2 tablespoons fresh orange juice
- 1 teaspoon of fresh lemon juice
- 2 tablespoons chopped fresh dill

#### Instructions

Preheat the air fryer to 350°F. Mix parsley, thyme, and 1/2 tsp salt. Brush salmon with oil and coat with herbs. Air fry two fillets at 350°F for 10 minutes; repeat with the rest. Meanwhile, mix fennel, coconut yogurt, garlic, orange juice, lemon juice, dill, and remaining salt. Serve salmon over fennel salad.

**Servings-2, Kcal- 713**
**Proteins- 51g, Fats- 47g, Carbs- 18g**

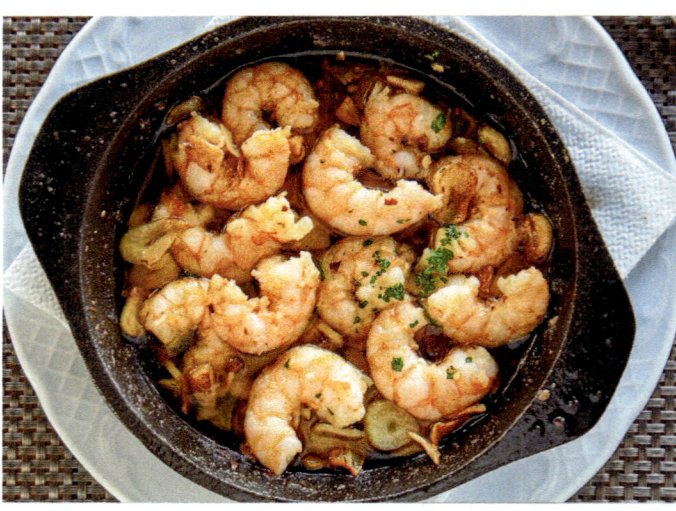

### Fiery Prawns

#### Ingredients

- Shrimp – raw - jumbo (1 lb.)
- Garlic powder (0.5 t.)
- Olive oil (2 tbsp.)
- Tabasco sauce (1 t.)
- Water (2 tbsp.)
- Dried parsley (0.5 t.)
- Red pepper flakes (1 t.)
- Onion salt (0.5 t.)
- Smoked paprika (0.5 t.)
- Oregano - dried (1 t.)
- Black pepper (0.5 t.)

#### Instructions

Discard the veins and shells from the shrimp. Mix all ingredients (except the shrimp) in a resealable plastic bag. Add the shrimp, shake to coat, and marinate in the fridge for 4-6 hours. Cook in a fryer until pink (10 minutes). Serve with your favorite side. For oven: Bake at 400°F for 10-12 minutes until the shrimp turn pink.

**Servings - 3, Calories: 194**
**Protein: 25 g | Carbs - 3g | Fat: 9 g**

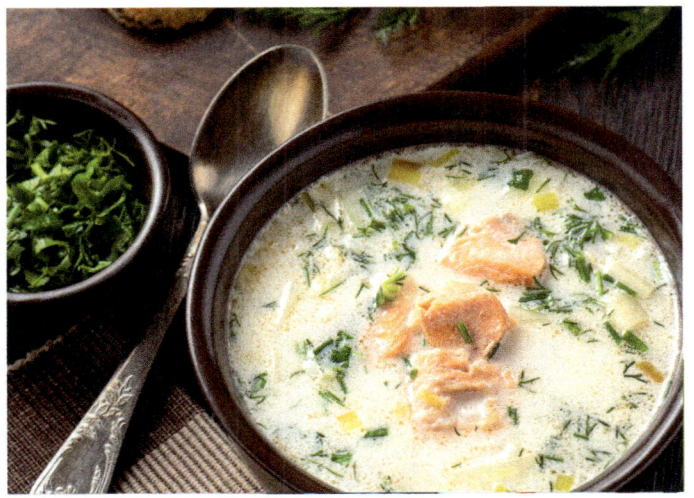

### Creamy leek and salmon soup

## Ingredients

- 2 tablespoons of avocado oil
- 2 tablespoons of dried thyme leaves
- 4 leeks, washed and cut
- 1 pound of salmon in small pieces
- 3 garlic cloves chopped
- 1 ¾ cups of coconut milk
- 6 cups of seafood or chicken broth
- Salt and pepper to taste

## Instructions

Heat avocado oil in a saucepan over medium heat. Sauté leeks and garlic until soft. Add broth, thyme, salt, and pepper; simmer for 15 minutes. Stir in salmon and coconut milk, cooking for 5-7 minutes until the salmon is tender. Serve!

**Servings - 2, Calories: 673**
**Protein: 33 g | Carbs: 32 g | Fat: 48g**

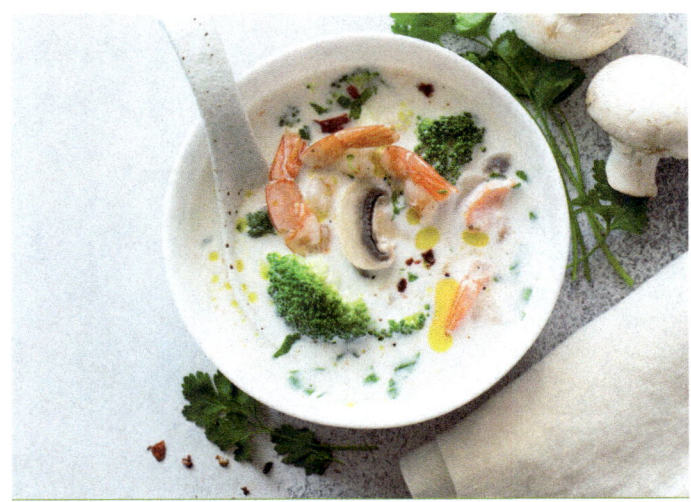

### Coconut soup with shrimp

## Ingredients

- **Broth:** 4 cups of chicken broth
- 1 cup fresh coriander
- 1.5 cups of fat coconut milk
- 3 or 4 dried thai peppers
- 1 organic lime
- 1 inch fresh galangal root
- Dried lemongrass, salt (1 teaspoon)
- **Soup:** 100 g raw wild caught shrimp
- 30 g red onion, chopped
- Coconut oil, fish sauce, cilantro (1 tbsp)
- 30 g mushrooms sliced
- Juice of 1 lime

## Instructions

Simmer the broth ingredients for 20 minutes, strain, and return to the pan. Bring to a boil, then add shrimp or chicken, fish sauce, onions, and mushrooms. Cook for 10 minutes until the meat is done. Stir in lime juice, garnish with cilantro, and serve.

**Servings - 1, Calories: 466**
**Protein: 30 g | Carbs: 21 g | Fat: 30 g**

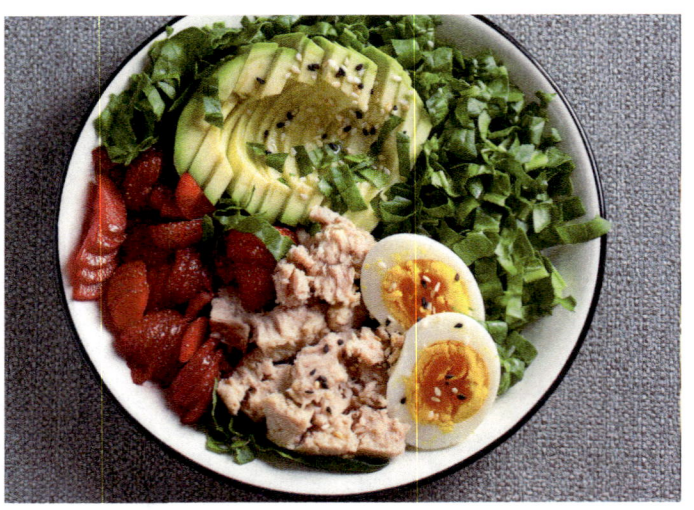

## Tuna and Strawberry Salad

### Ingredients

- 1 can (5 oz) tuna, drained
- 2 cups fresh spinach
- ½ cup strawberries, sliced
- ½ avocado, diced
- 1 boiled egg, sliced
- 1 tbsp olive oil
- 1 tbsp lemon juice
- Salt and pepper to taste

### Instructions

In a large bowl, layer spinach, tuna, strawberries, avocado, and boiled egg. Drizzle olive oil and lemon juice, then season with salt and pepper.

**Servings -1, Calories: 400**
**Protein: 35 g | Carbs: 15 g | Fat: 25 g**

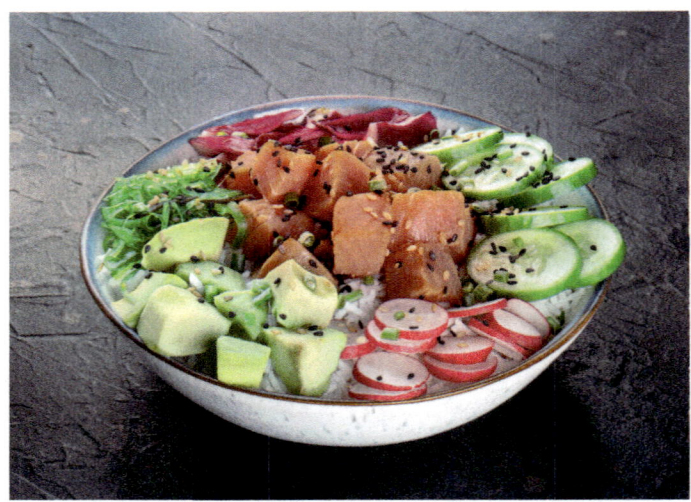

## Tuna Poke Bowl Recipe

### Ingredients

- 6 oz sushi-grade tuna (diced)
- ½ avocado (sliced)
- ½ cup cucumber (diced)
- ¼ cup wakame seaweed salad
- ¼ cup purple cabbage (shredded)
- 2 radishes (thinly sliced)
- 1 tsp sesame seeds
- 1 tbsp coconut aminos
- Sesame oil, rice vinegar (1 tsp)
- Grated ginger, garlic (½ tsp)
- ½ cup cooked jasmine rice (optional)

### Instructions

Whisk coconut aminos, sesame oil, rice vinegar, ginger, and garlic in a bowl. Add diced tuna, mix well, and let marinate for 10 minutes. In a serving bowl, arrange rice (if using), then top with tuna, avocado, cucumber, wakame, cabbage, and radishes. Sprinkle sesame seeds on top and serve immediately.

**Servings - 1, Calories: 577**
**Protein: 48 g| Carbs: 50 g | Fat: 20g**

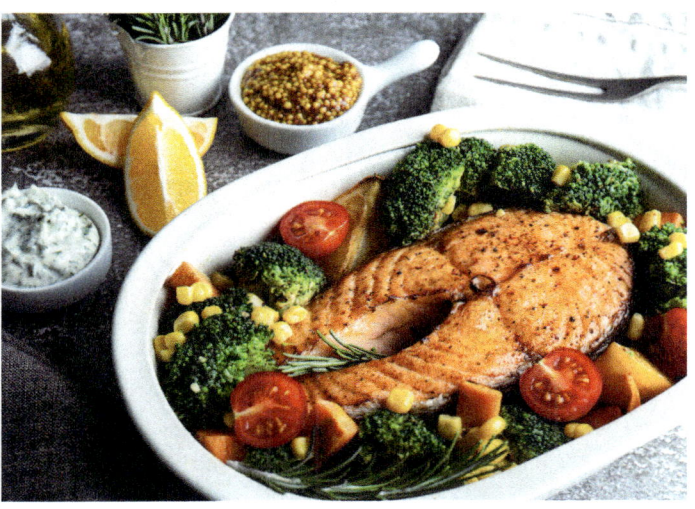

## Salmon with Carrots and Broccoli

### Ingredients

- 2 salmon steaks (6 oz each)
- 1 cup broccoli florets
- 1 cup carrot slices
- 2 tbsp olive oil
- 2 garlic cloves, minced
- ½ tsp turmeric
- ½ tsp sea salt
- ½ tsp black pepper
- ½ tsp dried thyme
- 1 tbsp lemon juice

### Instructions

Preheat the oven to 375°F (190°C). Place the salmon steaks on a baking sheet lined with parchment paper. Toss the broccoli and carrots with olive oil, garlic, turmeric, salt, pepper, and thyme, then spread them around the salmon. Drizzle lemon juice over everything. Bake for 15-18 minutes, or until the salmon is cooked through and flakes easily with a fork. Serve hot.

**Servings - 2, Calories: 550**
**Protein: 42 g | Carbs: -14g | Fat: 36 g**

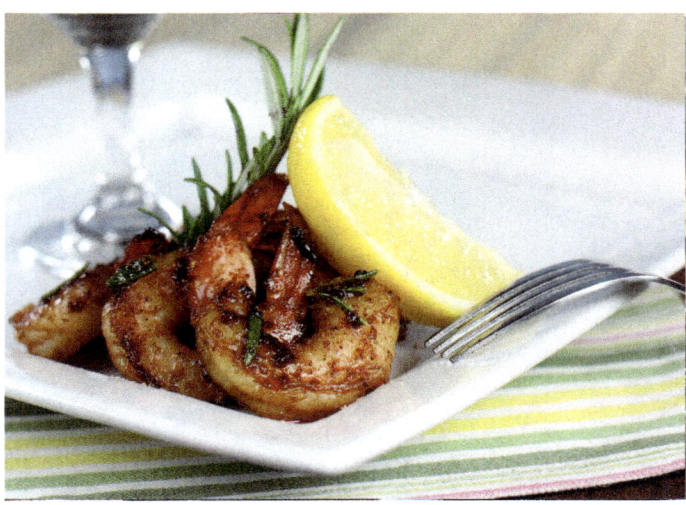

## Cajun Jumbo Shrimp

### Ingredients

- Shrimp - cleaned (1 lb.)
- Olive oil (1 tbsp.)
- Cajun seasoning (2 tbsp.)
- Black pepper (0.25 t.)
- Kosher salt (0.5 t.)

**Remainder of spices @ 1 t. each:**
- Dried thyme, Garlic powder, Paprika, Cayenne pepper or Chili powder, Onion powder

### Instructions

Preheat the oven to 370°F (188°C). Peel, devein, rinse, and dry the shrimp. Toss them with oil and seasonings, then spread them in a single layer on a baking sheet. Bake for 10-12 minutes, shaking halfway, until the shrimp are cooked. Serve hot. For the Air Fryer: Air fry shrimp at 370°F (188°C) for 8 minutes, shaking halfway until cooked.

**Servings - 4, Calories: 131**
**Protein: 22 g | Carbs: 2 g | Fat: 3 g**

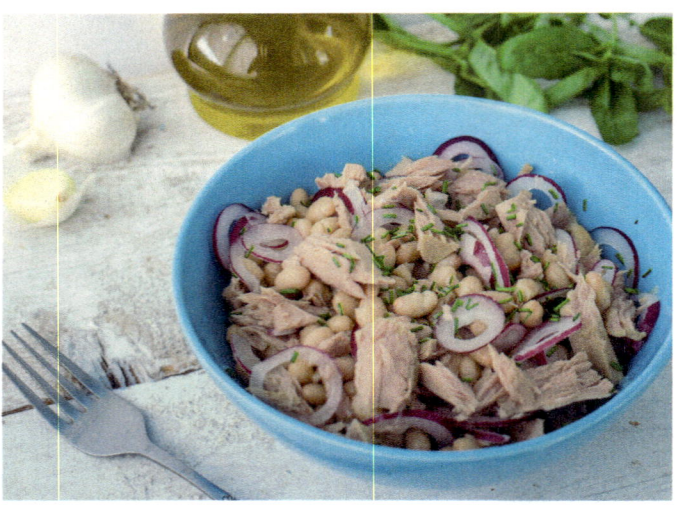

## Tuna and White Bean Salad

### Ingredients

- 2 cans (5 oz each) tuna in water, drained
- 1 can (15 oz) white beans, drained and rinsed
- 1/2 red onion, finely chopped
- 1/4 cup fresh parsley, chopped
- 2 tbsp olive oil
- 1 tbsp lemon juice
- Salt and pepper to taste

### Instructions

Combine tuna, white beans, red onion, and parsley in a large bowl. Drizzle with olive oil and lemon juice, season with salt and pepper, and toss everything together until well-mixed. Serve immediately or chill in the fridge for 30 minutes for the flavors to meld.

**Serving: 4, Calories: 290**
**Proteins: 22, Fats: 12, Carbs: 20**

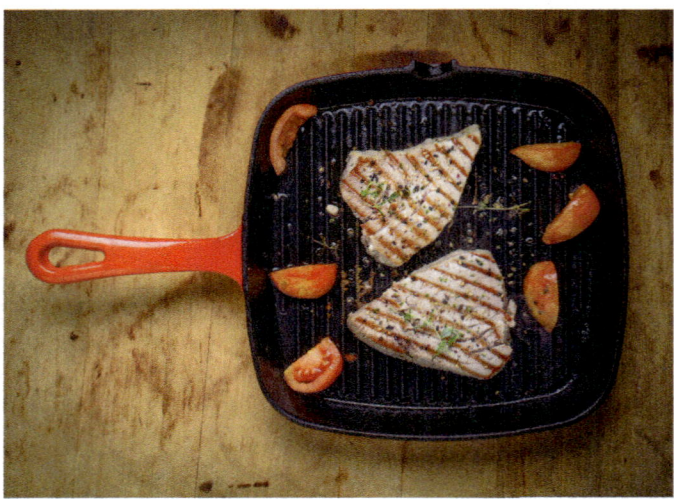

## Pan-Seared Tuna Steaks

### Ingredients

- 2 tuna steaks (about 6 ounces each)
- 2 tablespoons olive oil
- Salt and pepper to taste
- Optional: 1 teaspoon garlic powder, 1 teaspoon onion powder, 1 teaspoon dried thyme or rosemary

### Instructions

Season the tuna steaks with salt, pepper, garlic powder, onion powder, and dried thyme or rosemary if using. Heat olive oil in a skillet over medium-high heat until hot. Add the tuna steaks to the skillet. Sear the steaks for 2-3 minutes on each side for medium-rare, or adjust the time according to your preferred level of doneness. Remove from the skillet and let rest for a couple of minutes before serving. Serve hot.

**Servings-2, Kcal- 200**
**Proteins- 25g, Fats- 10g, Carbs- 1g**

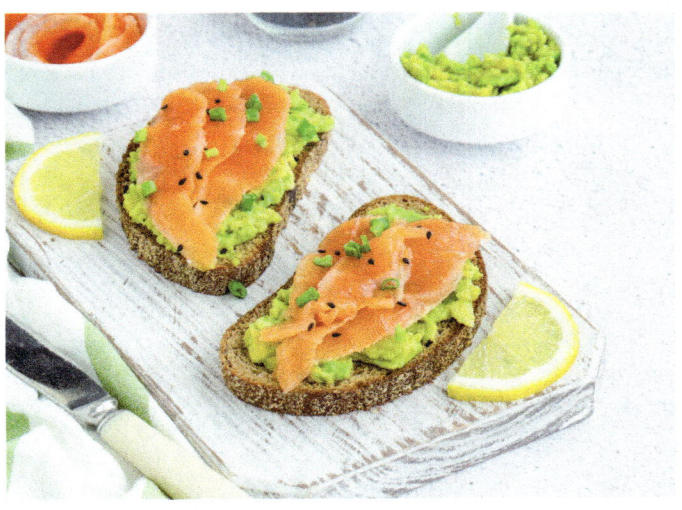 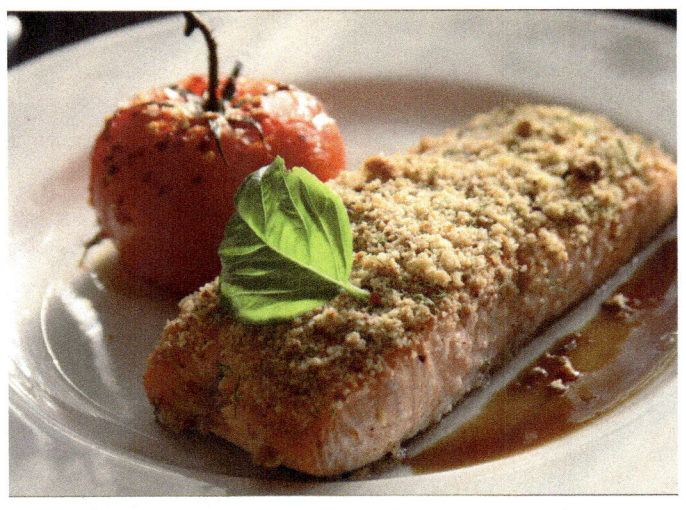

## Salmon and Avocado Toast

### Ingredients

- Two slices of whole-grain bread
- 4 oz smoked salmon
- One ripe avocado
- 1 tbsp lemon juice
- Fresh dill for garnish

### Instructions

Toast the bread. Mash the avocado with lemon juice and spread it on the toast. Top with smoked salmon and garnish with dill.

**Serving: 2, Calories: 210**
**Proteins: 10, Fats: 11, Carbs: 18**

## Walnut-Crusted Salmon

### Ingredients

- 2 salmon fillets
- 1/4 cup crushed walnuts
- 1 tbsp Dijon mustard
- 1 tbsp honey
- Salt and pepper to taste

### Instructions

Preheat the oven to 400°F (200°C). Mix Dijon mustard and honey, and brush onto the salmon. Press the crushed walnuts onto the salmon—season with salt and pepper. Bake for 12-15 minutes until the salmon is flaky. For the Air Fryer: Air fry at 400°F (200°C) for 8-10 minutes until the salmon is flaky.

**Serving: 1, Calories: 400**
**Proteins: 35, Fats: 25, Carbs: 10**

# VEGETARIAN

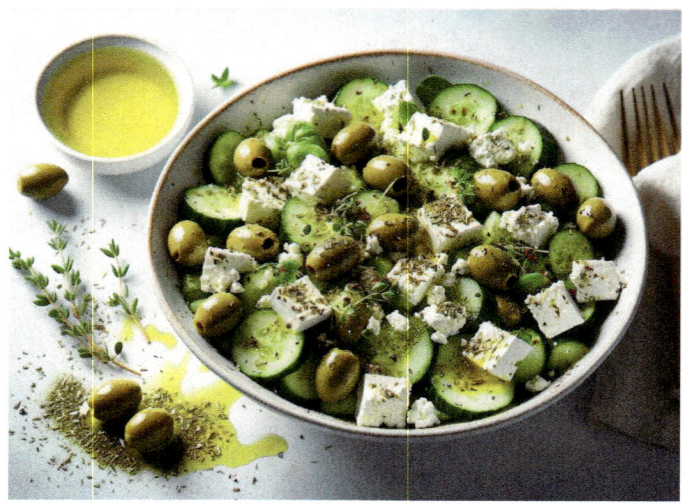

### Feta, and olive salad

## Ingredients

- Pinch of oregano, dried thyme
- 1 cup green olives
- 2 tablespoons of olive oil
- ½ cup feta
- 1 cup cucumber (chopped)

## Instructions

In a large bowl add all the ingredients. Mix well. Serve.

**Servings-1, Kcal- 620**
**Proteins- 3g, Fats- 64g, Carbs- 3g**

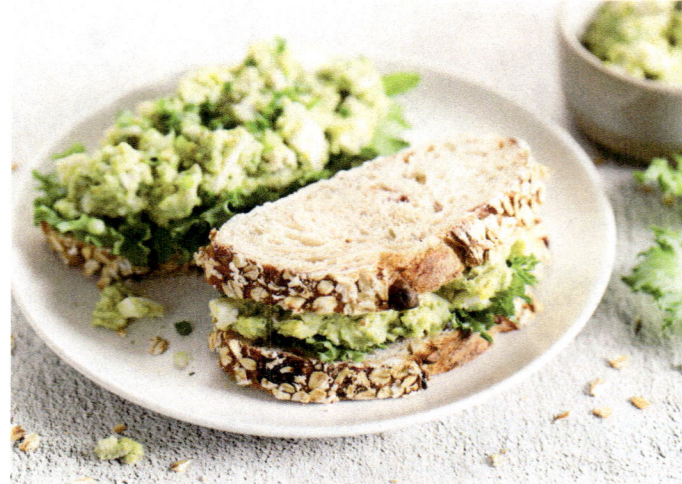

### Avocado and Chickpea Sandwich

## Ingredients

- 2 slices whole-grain bread
- 1/2 avocado mashed
- 1 tbsp lemon juice
- Salt and pepper
- 1/2 cup canned chickpeas, mashed
- Spinach leaves

## Instructions

Mix mashed avocado and chickpeas with lemon juice, salt, and pepper. Spread the mixture on one slice of bread. Add a layer of spinach leaves. Top with the second slice of bread and cut in half.

**Serving: 1, Calories: 350**
**Proteins: 12, Fats: 14, Carbs: 45**

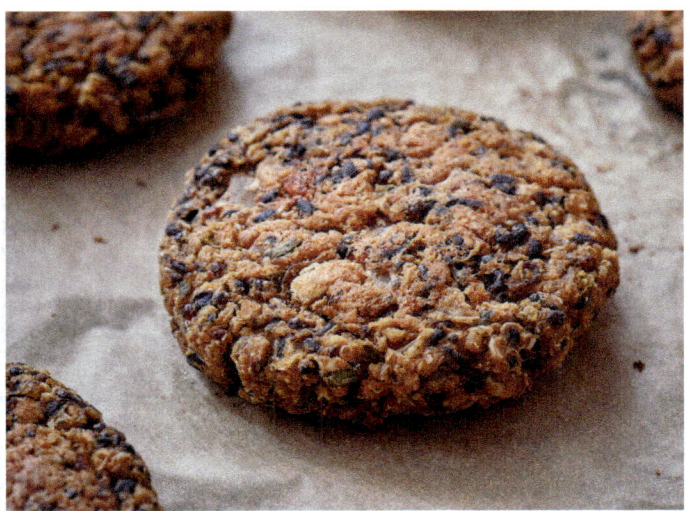

## Vegan Black Bean Burgers

### Ingredients

- 1 can black beans, rinsed and mashed
- 2 cloves garlic, minced
- ½ onion, finely chopped
- 1 tbsp chili powder
- 1 tbsp cumin
- ¼ cup almond flour or ground flaxseed
- 1 tbsp olive oil
- Salt to taste

### Instructions

Mash black beans in a bowl until mostly smooth. Stir in garlic, onion, chili powder, cumin, ground flaxseed/ almond flour, and salt. Mix well until combined—heat olive oil in a skillet over medium heat. Shape the mixture into small patties and cook for 3-4 minutes per side until crispy.

**Serving: 4, Calories: 230**
**Proteins: 12, Fats: 2, Carbs: 44**

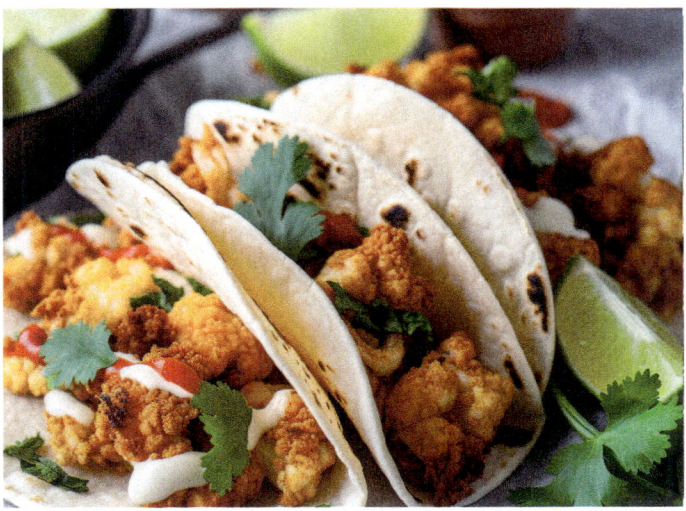

## Cauliflower Tacos

### Ingredients

- Cauliflower, cut into florets (1 head)
- Olive oil (2 tablespoons)
- Chili powder (1 teaspoon)
- Cumin, Garlic powder (½ teaspoon)
- Salt and pepper, to taste

**For the Tacos:**
- Small whole grain tortillas ( 8 )
- Shredded lettuce (1 cup)
- Red onion, Cilantro (¼ cup)
- Lime wedges, for serving

### Instructions

Preheat the oven to 400°F (200°C). Toss the cauliflower with oil and spices and roast for 25-30 minutes, flipping halfway. Fill the warm tortillas with cauliflower, lettuce, onion, cilantro. For the Air Fryer: Air fry at 375°F (190°C) for 15 - 18 minutes.

**Servings-2, Calories: 465**
**Carbs: 75 g, Fat: 20 g, Protein: 9 g**

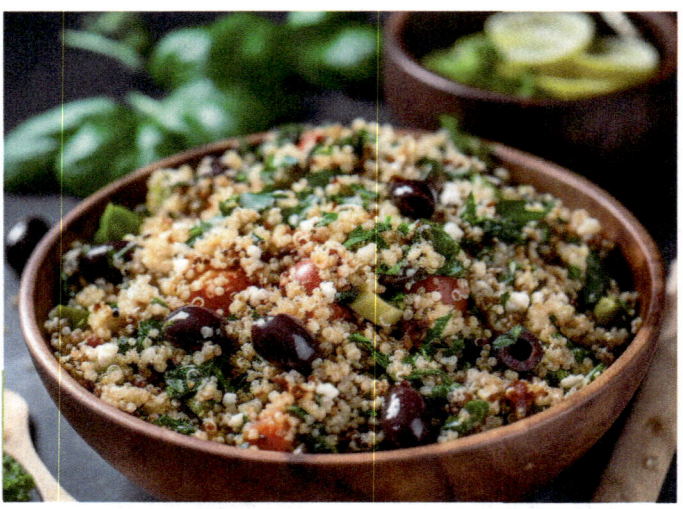

## Mediterranean Quinoa Salad

### Ingredients

- Quinoa (1 cup)
- Water (2 cups)
- Salt and pepper, to taste
- Cucumbers, Cherry tomatoes, (1 cup)
- Red onion, Parsley chopped (½ cup)
- Kalamata olives, sliced (¼ cup)
- Extra-virgin olive oil (3 tablespoons)
- Lemon juice (2 tablespoons)
- Garlic, minced (1 clove)
- Dried oregano (1 teaspoon)

### Instructions

Preheat the oven to 350°F. Cook the quinoa with salt and let it cool. Mix the quinoa, cucumbers, tomatoes, onion, parsley, and olives. Whisk the oil, garlic, lemon, oregano, salt, and pepper; drizzle over the salad. Bake for 5 minutes, mix, and serve. For the Air Fryer: Air fry at 350°F for 2-3 minutes, mix, and serve.

**Servings-2, Calories: 367**
**Carbs: 42 g, Fat: 24 g, Protein: 8 g**

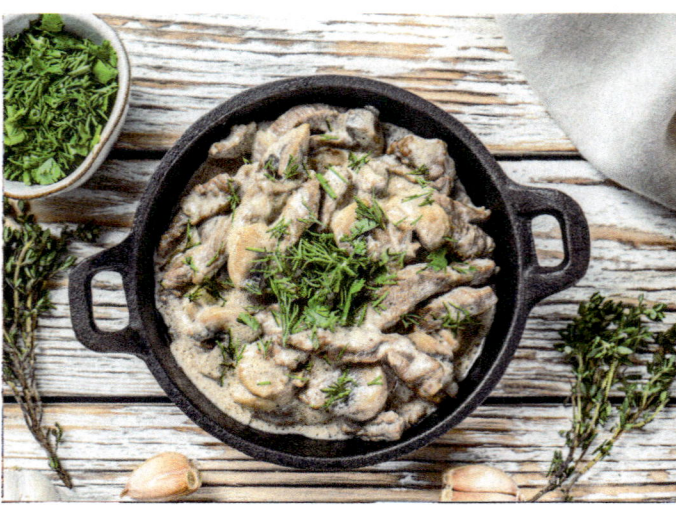

## Mushroom Stroganoff

### Ingredients

- 1 tablespoon olive oil
- 1 medium onion, finely chopped
- 3 cloves garlic, minced
- 1 pound (450g) mushrooms, sliced
- Vegetable broth, Coconut milk (1 cup)
- 2 tablespoons of coconut aminos
- 2 tablespoons almond flour
- 1 tbsp nutritional yeast (optional)
- 1 tablespoon lemon juice
- Salt and pepper, to taste
- Fresh parsley, chopped (for garnish)

### Instructions

Heat olive oil in a skillet. Sauté onion for 5 minutes, add garlic for 1-2 minutes, then mushrooms until golden (8-10 minutes). Stir in flour, then gradually add vegetable broth until thickened. Mix in coconut milk, coconut aminos, and nutritional yeast (if using). Simmer for 5-7 minutes, then add lemon juice, season, and garnish with parsley.

**Servings-4, Calories: 100**
**Carbs: 7 g, Fat: 8 g, Protein: 3 g**

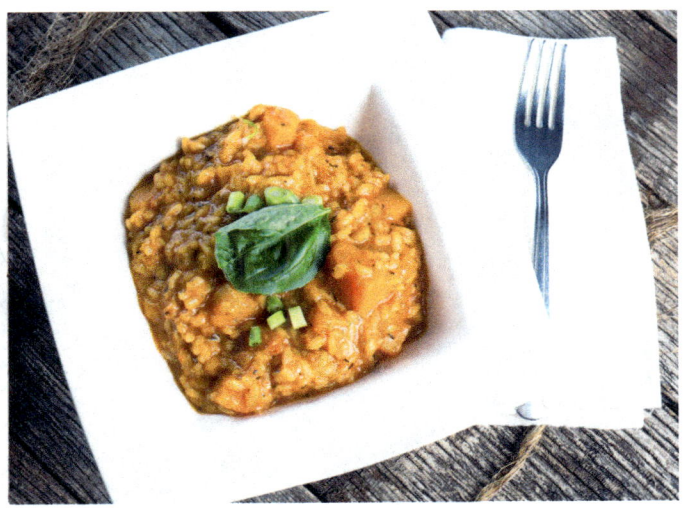

## Butternut Squash Risotto

### Ingredients

- 1 medium butternut squash, cubed
- 1 tbsp olive oil
- 1 small onion, finely chopped
- 2 cloves garlic, minced
- 1 cup quinoa (or cauliflower rice for low-carb)
- 4 cups vegetable broth (low-sodium)
- ½ tsp turmeric
- ½ tsp dried thyme
- 2 tbsp lemon juice
- ½ cup nutritional yeast
- Salt and pepper to taste
- Fresh parsley, chopped (for garnish)

### Instructions

Heat olive oil, sauté onion, garlic, butternut squash, and cook for 5 minutes. Stir in quinoa, turmeric, thyme, lemon juice, and broth. Simmer for 15–20 minutes until tender. Mix in nutritional yeast, season, and garnish with parsley.

**Servings-1, Kcal- 622**
**Proteins- 26g, Fats- 19g, Carbs- 95g**

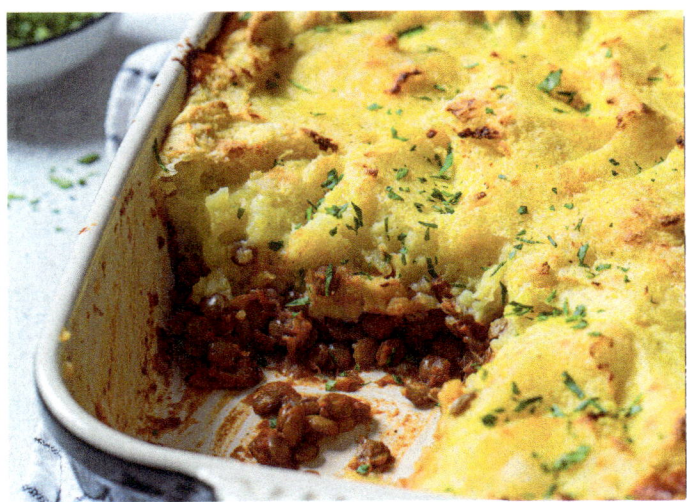

## Vegan Shepherd's Pie

### Ingredients

- 1 tbsp olive oil
- 1 onion, chopped
- 2 cloves garlic, minced
- 2 carrots, diced
- 1 tbsp tomato paste
- 1 cup vegetable broth
- 1.5 cups cooked lentils
- ½ tsp turmeric
- Salt and pepper to taste
- 2 large sweet potatoes, peeled
- ¼ cup plant-based milk
- 2 tbsp olive oil

### Instructions

Sauté onion, garlic, and carrots in olive oil. Add tomato paste, broth, lentils, turmeric, salt, and pepper; simmer until thick. Boil sweet potatoes and mash with plant-based milk and olive oil. Layer lentil mixture in a baking dish, top with mashed sweet potatoes, and bake at 375°F for 20 minutes.

**Serving: 2, Calories: 512**
**Proteins: 16, Fats: 22, Carbs: 68**

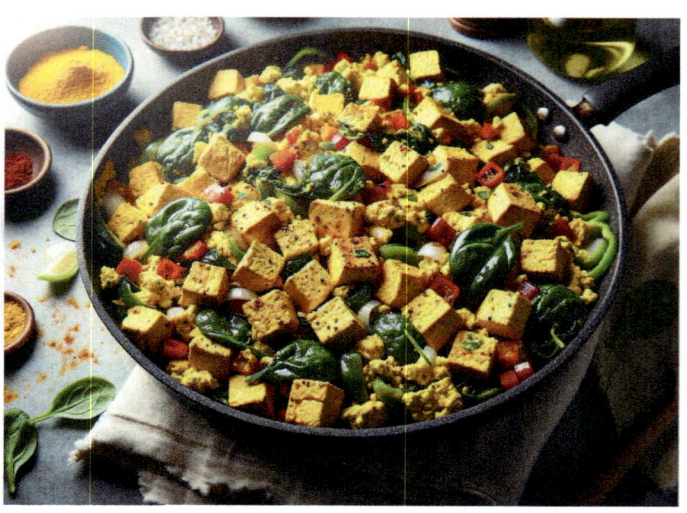
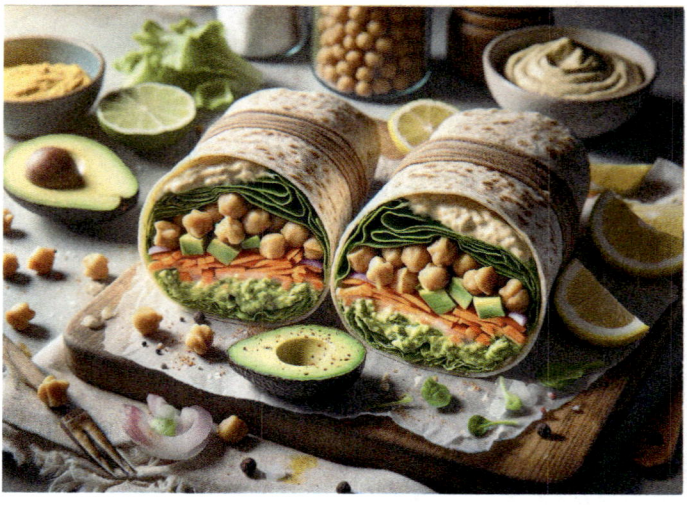

## Protein-Packed Tofu Scramble

### Ingredients

- 1/2 block firm tofu, crumbled
- 1 tablespoon olive oil
- 1/2 teaspoon turmeric
- 1/2 cup diced bell pepper
- 1/4 cup diced onion
- 1 cup spinach leaves
- Salt and pepper to taste
- 1 tbsp nutritional yeast

### Instructions

Heat olive oil in a pan over medium heat. Add turmeric, bell pepper, and onion; sauté until soft. Add crumbled tofu and cook for 5-7 minutes, stirring occasionally. Stir in spinach until wilted. Season with salt, pepper, and nutritional yeast.

**Serving: 1, Calories: 250**
**Proteins: 18, Fats: 16, Carbs: 10**

## Chickpea and Avocado Wrap

### Ingredients

- Whole-grain wraps: 4
- Canned chickpeas: 1 can (15 oz)
- Ripe avocado: 1 large, mashed
- Lettuce: 4 large leaves (1 per wrap)
- Shredded carrots: 1 cup
- Hummus: 4 tablespoons (1 tablespoon per wrap)
- Lemon juice: 1 tablespoon
- Salt and pepper: To taste

### Instructions

Mash the avocado with lemon juice, salt, and pepper. Spread hummus over the wraps and top with lettuce, shredded carrots, chickpeas, and mashed avocado. Roll up the wraps tightly and cut them in half.

**Serving: 4, Calories: 345**
**Proteins: 12, Fats: 13, Carbs: 47**

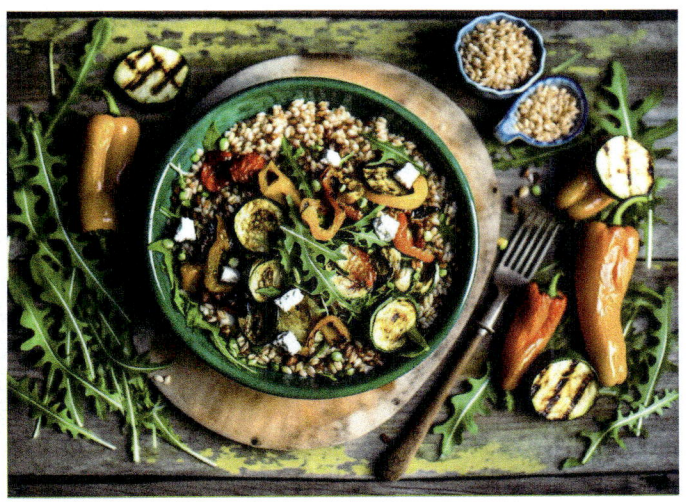

## Roasted Veggie and Farro Bowl

### Ingredients

- Assorted vegetables (zucchini, bell peppers, onions): 4 cups, chopped
- Farro: 1 cup, uncooked
- Olive oil: 2 tablespoons
- Balsamic vinegar: 2 tablespoons
- Feta cheese: 1/2 cup, crumbled
- Arugula: 2 cups
- Salt: To taste
- Pepper: To taste

### Instructions

Toss the vegetables in olive oil, balsamic vinegar, salt, and pepper, and roast until tender. Cook farro according to package directions. Assemble the bowl with a bed of arugula, farro, roasted veggies, and crumbled feta cheese.

**Serving: 4, Calories: 285**
**Proteins: 9, Fats: 12, Carbs: 38**

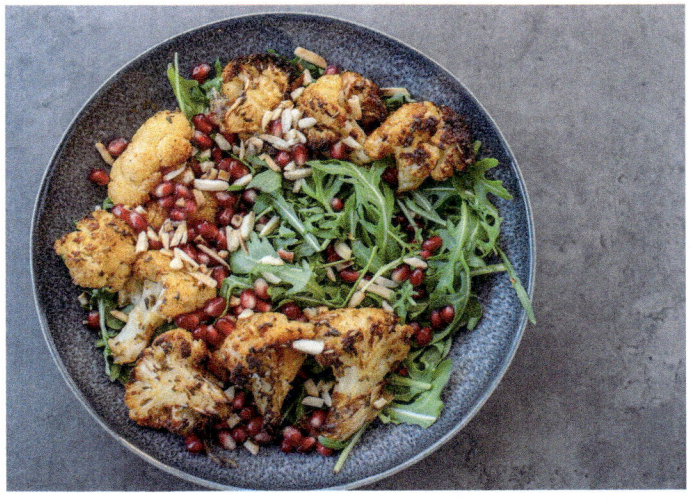

## Roasted Cauliflower Salad

### Ingredients

- 1 head of cauliflower, cut into florets
- 1 tbsp olive oil
- 1/2 tsp turmeric
- Salt and pepper to taste
- 2 cups mixed greens
- 1 tbsp pumpkin seeds
- 1/4 cup pomegranate seeds

### Instructions

Preheat the oven to 425°F (220°C). Toss the cauliflower with olive oil, turmeric, salt, and pepper. Roast for 25 minutes. Arrange mixed greens on a plate and top with the roasted cauliflower, pomegranate, and pumpkin seeds. For the Air Fryer, Air fry at 375°F (190°C) for 12-15 minutes, shaking halfway.

**Serving: 1, Calories: 151**
**Proteins: 5, Fats: 7, Carbs: 18**

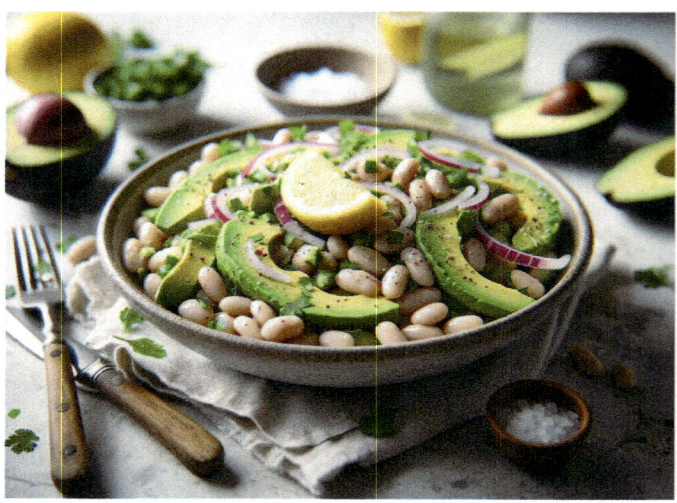

## Avocado and White Bean Salad

### Ingredients

- 1 can (15 oz) white beans (rinsed)
- 1 ripe avocado, diced
- 1/4 red onion, thinly sliced
- 1/4 cup fresh cilantro, chopped
- 2 tablespoons olive oil
- 1 tablespoon lemon juice
- 1 teaspoon garlic powder
- 1/2 teaspoon ground cumin
- Salt and pepper, to taste

### Instructions

Combine the white beans, diced avocado, red onion, and cilantro in a large bowl. In a small bowl, whisk together the olive oil, lemon juice, garlic powder, cumin, salt, and pepper. Pour the dressing over the salad and gently toss to combine. Serve immediately or refrigerate for 30 minutes to allow the flavors to meld.

**Serving: 2, Calories: 370**
**Proteins: 9, Fats: 23, Carbs: 34**

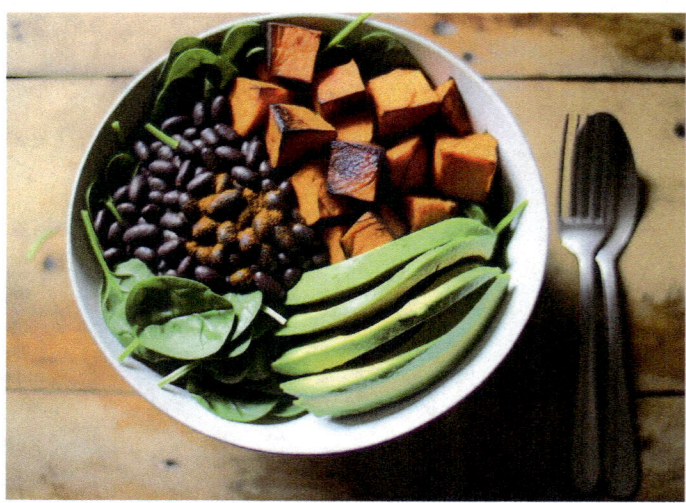

## Sweet Potato & Black Bean Bowl

### Ingredients

- 1 medium sweet potato, cubed
- 1/2 cup black beans, cooked
- 1/2 avocado, sliced
- 1 cup spinach leaves
- 1 tbsp olive oil
- 1/2 tsp ground cumin
- Salt and pepper to taste
- Lime juice for dressing

### Instructions

Roast sweet potato cubes with olive oil, cumin, salt, and pepper at 400°F (200°C) for 25 minutes. Assemble the bowl with spinach leaves, roasted sweet potato, black beans, and avocado. Drizzle with fresh lime juice before serving.

**Serving: 1, Calories: 320**
**Proteins: 8, Fats: 15, Carbs: 40**

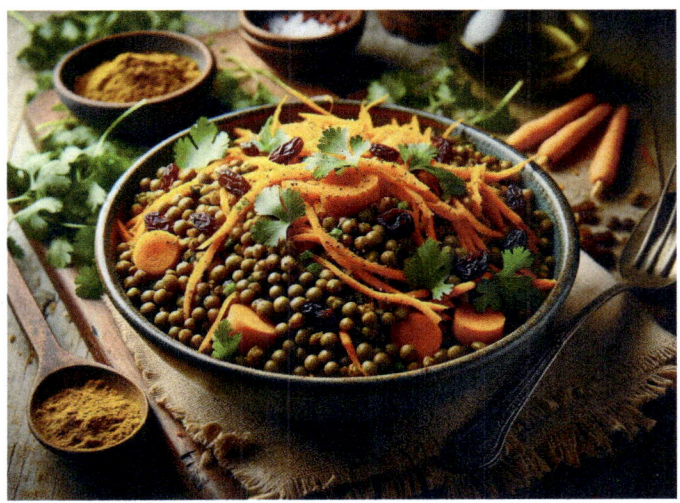

## Lentil & Carrot Salad

### Ingredients

- 1 cup cooked lentils
- 1 cup grated carrots
- 1/4 cup raisins
- 1/2 tsp curry powder
- 1 tbsp olive oil
- 1 tbsp apple cider vinegar
- Salt to taste
- Fresh cilantro for garnish

### Instructions

In a bowl, mix lentils, carrots, and raisins. Whisk together olive oil, apple cider vinegar, curry powder, and salt. Pour dressing over salad and toss to combine. Garnish with cilantro before serving.

**Serving: 1, Calories: 300**
**Proteins: 12, Fats: 7, Carbs: 50**

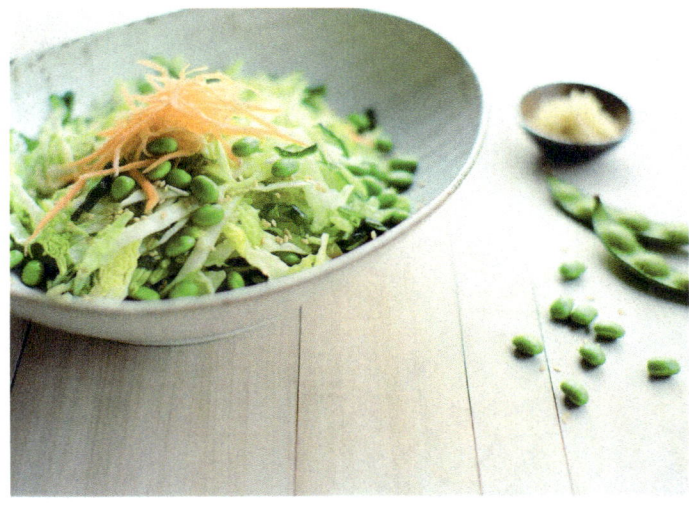

## Asian Cabbage and edamame Salad

### Ingredients

- 2 cups shredded cabbage
- 1 cup edamame, cooked
- 1 carrot, julienned
- 1 tbsp sesame oil
- 1 tbsp soy sauce
- 1 tsp grated ginger
- 1 tbsp sesame seeds

### Instructions

In a large bowl, combine cabbage, edamame, and carrot. Whisk together sesame oil, soy sauce, and ginger in a small bowl. Toss the salad with the dressing and sprinkle with sesame seeds.

**Serving: 1, Calories: 220**
**Proteins: 11, Fats: 14, Carbs: 15**

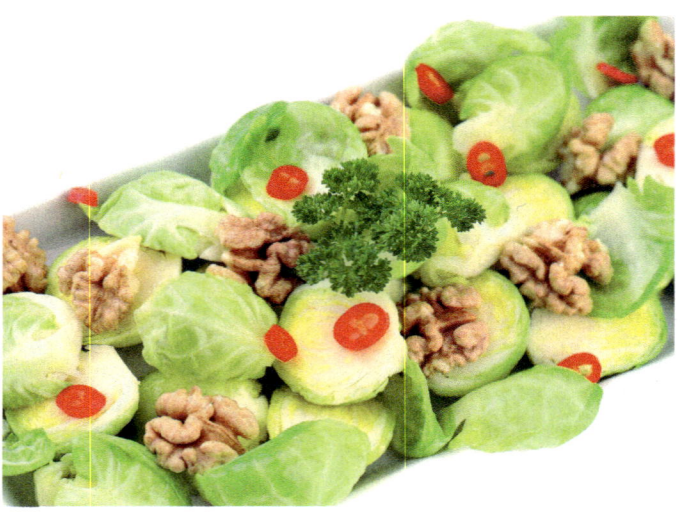

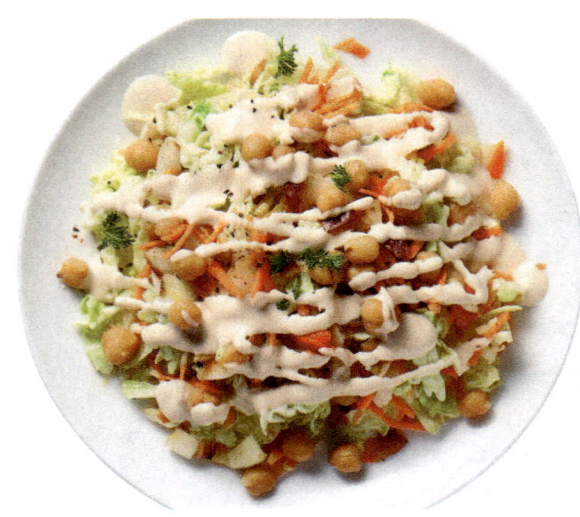

## Sprouts and Walnut Salad

### Ingredients

- Brussels sprouts, thinly sliced (1 pound)
- Walnuts, toasted, chopped (1/2 cup)
- Extra-virgin Olive oil (2 tablespoons)
- Balsamic Vinegar (2 tablespoons)
- Cranberries dried (1/4 cup)
- Salt and Pepper, to taste

### Instructions

Combine Brussels sprouts, walnuts, and cranberries in a bowl. Whisk the olive oil with balsamic vinegar in a separate bowl. Drizzle the dressing over the salad ingredients. Gently mix the salad with the dressing to ensure it is well coated. Season with salt and pepper to taste. Serve!

**Serving: 4, Calories: 210**
**Proteins: 5, Fats: 15, Carbs: 16**

## Cabbage and Chickpea Salad

### Ingredients

- Green cabbage shredded (4 cups)
- Chickpeas (1 can/15 oz)
- Carrots, grated (2)
- Fresh parsley, chopped 1/4 cup
- Tahini (1/4 cup)
- Juice of (1 lemon)
- Extra-Virgin Olive oil (2 tablespoons)
- Garlic, minced (1 clove )
- Salt and pepper, to taste

### Instructions

Combine the shredded cabbage, chickpeas, grated carrots, and chopped fresh parsley in a bowl. Mix extra-virgin olive oil with the tahini, lemon juice, and minced garlic in a separate bowl. Season with salt and pepper to taste. Adjust the dressing to your desired consistency by adding water if needed. Pour the dressing over the salad and give it a gentle toss until everything is coated in it. Taste and adjust the seasoning if needed. Serve!

**Serving: 1, Calories: 285**
**Proteins: 10, Fats: 13, Carbs: 33**

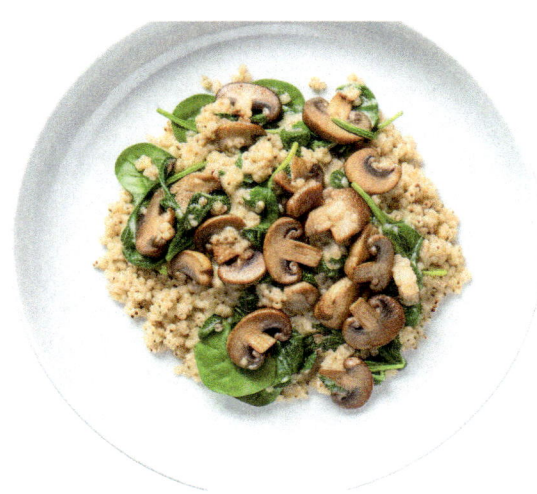
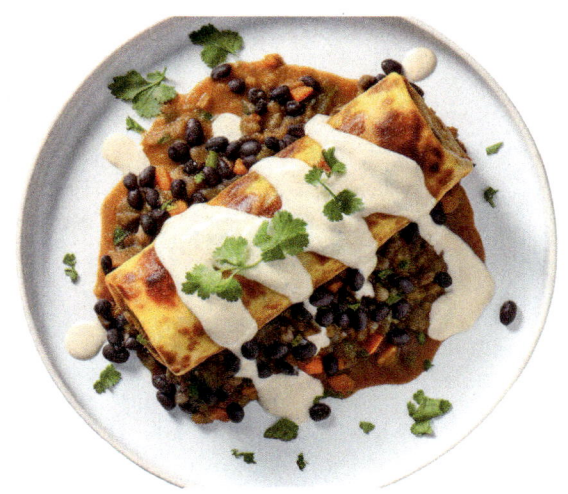

## Mushroom & Spinach Quinoa Pilaf

### Ingredients

- Vegetable broth (2 cups low-sodium)
- Quinoa, rinsed and drained (1 cup)
- Mushrooms, sliced (8 oz/225g)
- Fresh spinach leaves (2 cups)
- Dried thyme (1 teaspoon)
- Garlic cloves, minced (2)
- Salt and pepper, to taste
- Olive oil (2 tablespoons)
- Lemon zest (garnish)
- Onion, chopped (1)

### Instructions

Heat olive oil in a skillet over medium heat. Sauté onion, garlic, and mushrooms for 5 minutes. Add rinsed quinoa, toast briefly, then pour vegetable broth and thyme. Season with salt and pepper, bring to a boil, then simmer for 15-20 minutes until quinoa is cooked. Stir in spinach and cook for 2-3 minutes. Adjust seasoning, garnish with lemon zest.

**Serving: 4, Calories: 235**
**Proteins: 6, Fats: 7, Carbs: 33**

## Sweet Potato and Black BeanEnchilada

### Ingredients

- Olive oil ( 1 tablespoon)
- Garlic cloves, minced (2)
- Ground cumin (1 teaspoon)
- Chili powder (1/2 teaspoon)
- Onion, finely chopped (1 small)
- Fresh spinach, chopped (1 cup)
- Whole grain or corn tortillas (8)
- Turmeric powder (1/4 teaspoon)
- Black beans, rinsed (1 can/ 15 oz)
- Enchilada sauce (2 cups low sodium)
- Sweet potatoes, peeled and diced (2)
- Salt to taste, Fresh cilantro (garnish)

### Instructions

Preheat the oven to 375°F (190°C). Mash the boiled sweet potatoes. Sauté the onions, garlic, black beans, spinach, and spices. Mix with the sweet potatoes. Fill the tortillas, roll them, and place them in a sauced baking dish. Top with more sauce, cover, and bake for 20-25 minutes. Garnish with cilantro and serve.

**Serving: 4, Calories: 345**
**Proteins: 10, Fats: 9, Carbs: 50**

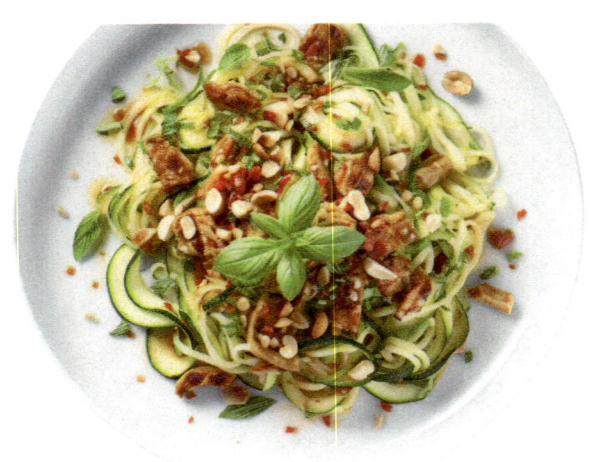
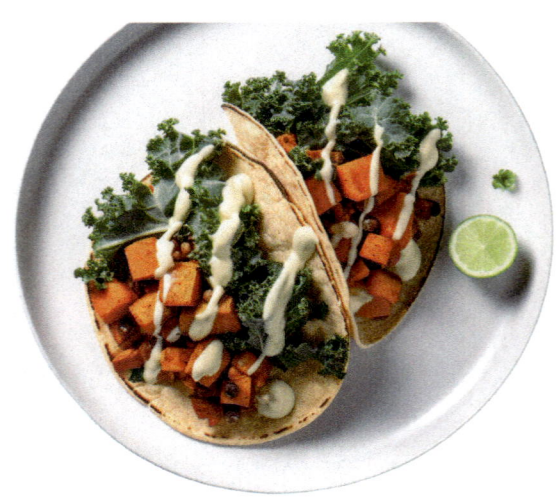

## Zucchini Noodle Pad Thai

### Ingredients
- Zucchinis, spiralized into noodles (4)
- Raw peanuts, chopped (1/4 cup)
- Olive oil or coconut oil (1 tablespoon)
- Green onions, Garlic cloves (2)
- Fresh cilantro (garnish)
- Carrot, Lime (1)

**For the sauce:**
- Maple syrup, Rice vinegar (1 tbsp)
- Chili flakes (1/2 teaspoon optional)
- Peanut butter, Tamari (2 tablespoons)
- Ginger grated, Sesame oil (1 tsp)

### Instructions
Prepare zucchini noodles. Whisk sauce ingredients until smooth. Heat oil in a skillet over medium heat. Sauté white green onions, garlic, and carrot for 3-4 minutes. Add zucchini noodles and stir-fry for 2-3 minutes. Mix in sauce and heat through. Garnish with green onion tops, peanuts, cilantro, and lime wedges.

**Serving: 4, Calories: 215**
**Proteins: 8, Fats: 14, Carbs: 21**

## Sweet Potato and Kale Tacos

### Ingredients
- Sweet potatoes, peeled and diced (2)
- Black beans, rinsed (1 can/ 15 oz)
- Kale, chopped (2 cups)
- Whole grain (8 small)
- Chili powder (1/4 teaspoon optional)
- Sea salt and black pepper, to taste
- Cilantro, chopped (1/4 cup)
- Olive oil (2 tablespoons)
- Turmeric (1/2 teaspoon)
- Cumin (1 teaspoon)
- Lime (1)

### Instructions
Preheat oven to 400°F (204°C) and bake sweet potatoes in olive oil for 20-25 minutes. Sauté kale, then add black beans, cumin, turmeric, chili powder, salt, and pepper. Stir in roasted sweet potatoes. Warm tortillas and fill with the mixture. Serve with lime and ranch.

**Serving: 4, Calories: 325**
**Proteins: 10, Fats: 13, Carbs: 46**

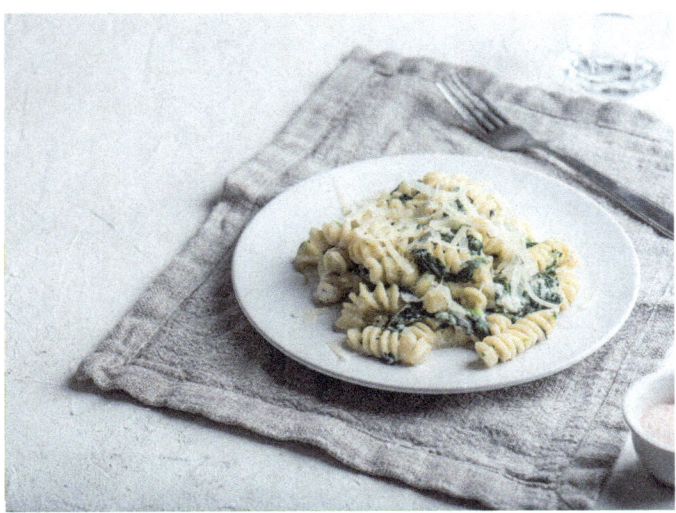

## Creamy Spinach & Artichoke Pasta

### Ingredients

- 340 g chickpea pasta
- 1 tbsp olive oil
- 3 cloves garlic, minced
- 1 cup canned artichoke hearts,
- 4 cups fresh spinach, chopped
- 1 ½ cups plant based milk
- 1 cup raw cashews (soaked in water )
- 3 tbsp nutritional yeast
- 1 tbsp lemon juice
- 1 tsp onion powder
- Salt, Black pepper (½ tsp)

### Instructions

Cook pasta, reserving ½ cup of water. Blend cashews, plant-based milk, nutritional yeast, lemon juice, and seasonings until smooth. Sauté garlic, artichoke hearts, and spinach in vegan butter or oil. Add sauce, stir in pasta.

**Serving: 4, Calories: 602**
**Proteins: 29, Fats: 24, Carbs: 70**

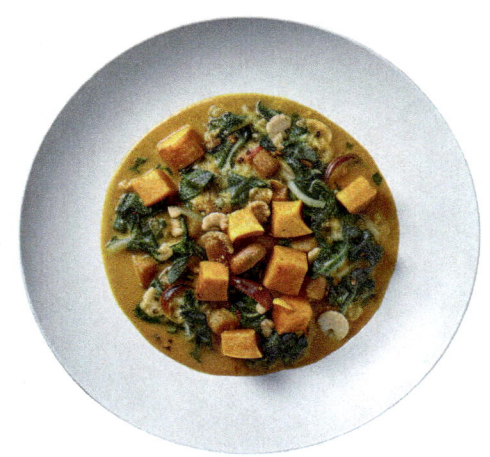

## Pumpkin and Spinach Curry

### Ingredients

- Cumin, Coriander (1 teaspoon)
- Turmeric (2 teaspoons)
- Fresh cilantro, (garnish)
- Garlic cloves , minced (3)
- Spinach fresh, Pumpkin (2 cups)
- Onion, Ginger (1 medium)
- Coconut milk (1 can/ 14 oz full-fat)
- Sea salt and black pepper, to taste
- Chili powder (1/2 teaspoon optional)
- Coconut oil or olive oil (2 tbsp)
- Lemon or lime juice (1 tbsp garnish)

### Instructions

Heat olive oil in a skillet, sauté onions, garlic, and ginger until caramelized. Add turmeric, cumin, coriander, and chili powder; cook until fragrant. Stir in pumpkin, coat with spices, add coconut milk, and simmer for 15-20 minutes until tender. Add spinach, cook until wilted, then season with salt, pepper, and lemon juice. Garnish with cilantro.

**Serving: 4, Calories: 255**
**Proteins: 5, Fats: 23, Carbs: 14**

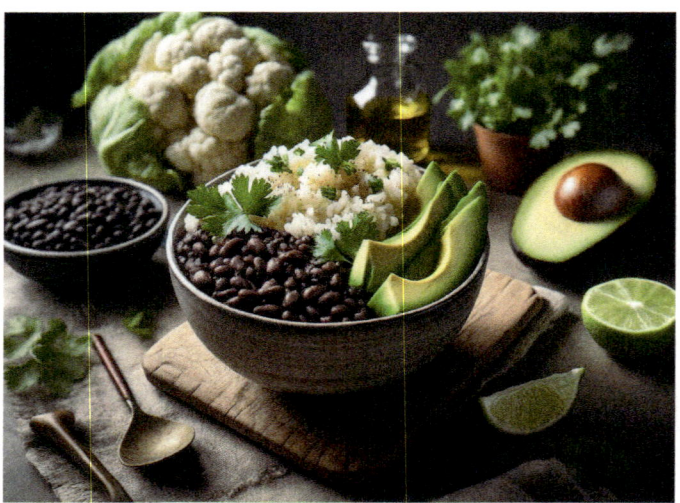

## Cauliflower Rice & Black Bean Bowl

### Ingredients

- 1 cup cauliflower rice
- ½ cup dried black beans
- ½ avocado, sliced
- Fresh cilantro, chopped
- Juice of 1 lime
- Sea salt to taste

### Instructions

Rinse and soak the dried black beans overnight, then drain and rinse again. In a pot, cover the beans with fresh water and bring to a boil. Then, reduce to a simmer and cook for 60–90 minutes until tender, adding salt in the last 10 minutes. Meanwhile, steam or sauté the cauliflower rice for 3–5 minutes until tender. To assemble, serve the cauliflower rice topped with black beans, avocado slices, fresh cilantro, and a squeeze of lime juice. Enjoy!

**Servings-1, Kcal- 350**
**Proteins- 15g, Fats- 15g, Carbs- 45**

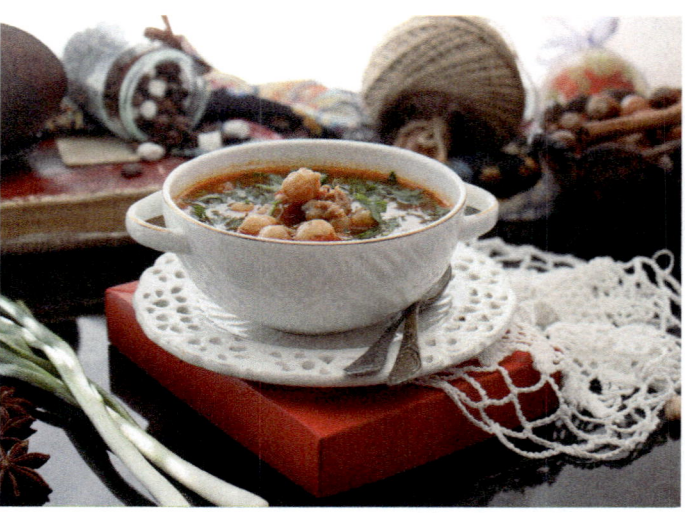

## Moroccan Chickpea Soup

### Ingredients

- 1/2 cup chickpeas
- 1/4 cup diced onions
- 1/2 tsp cumin
- 1/2 tsp coriander
- Vegetable broth

### Instructions

Sauté onions in a pot over medium heat for 3-4 minutes until soft. Add cumin and coriander, stirring for 30 seconds until fragrant. Add chickpeas and vegetable broth (enough to cover). Bring to a boil, then reduce heat and simmer for 20-25 minutes until flavors meld. Serve warm.

**Servings-1, Kcal- 250**
**Proteins- 12g, Fats- 4g, Carbs- 40**

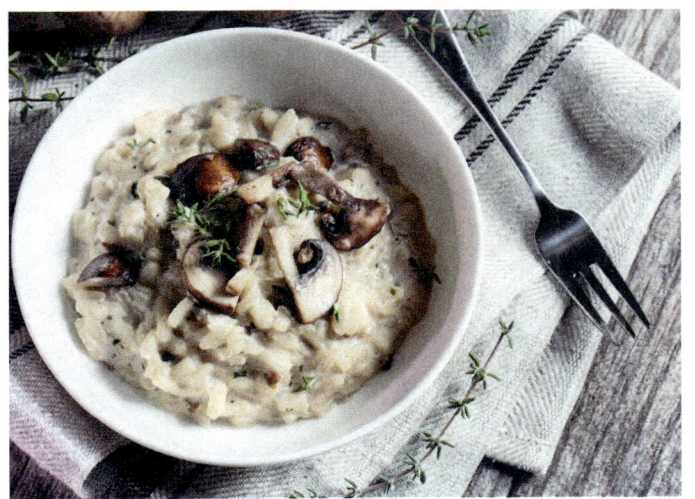

### Mushroom Risotto

## Ingredients

- 1 cup quinoa (or cauliflower rice for low-carb)
- 2 tbsp olive oil
- 1 small onion, finely chopped
- 3 cloves garlic, minced
- 8 oz (225 g) mushrooms, sliced
- 4 cups vegetable broth, warmed
- 2 tbsp nutritional yeast
- 1/2 tsp turmeric
- 1/4 tsp black pepper
- Salt to taste
- Fresh parsley, chopped (for garnish)

## Instructions

Heat olive oil in a pan over medium heat. Sauté onion and garlic until soft. Add mushrooms and cook until browned. Stir in quinoa, turmeric, and black pepper. Gradually pour in warm broth, stirring until absorbed. Cook until quinoa is tender. Stir in nutritional yeast, season with salt, and garnish with parsley.

**Serving: 2, Calories: 418**
**Proteins: 24, Fats: 17, Carbs: 48**

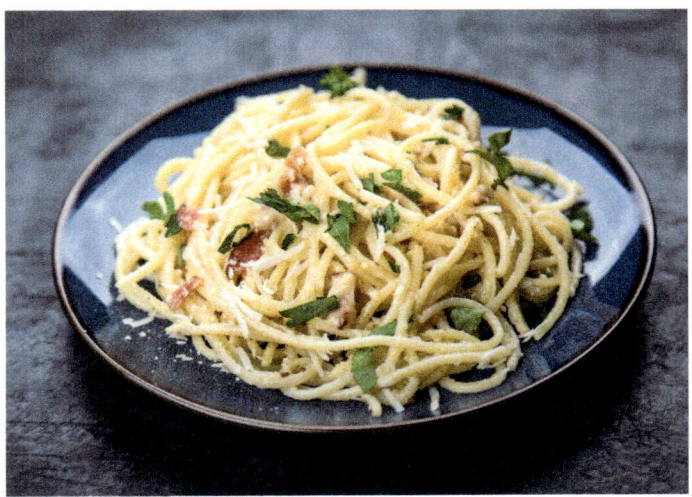

### Vegan Spaghetti Carbonara

## Ingredients

- 12 oz whole grain spaghetti
- 2 tbsp olive oil
- 1 large onion, finely chopped
- 3 garlic cloves, minced
- 1 cup smoked tofu, diced
- 1 cup cashews, soaked and drained
- 1 cup unsweetened almond milk
- 1/4 cup nutritional yeast
- 1 tbsp lemon juice
- 1 tbsp coconut aminos
- 1/2 tsp turmeric
- Salt and pepper to taste
- Fresh parsley, chopped (for garnish)

## Instructions

Cook spaghetti. Sauté onion, garlic, and tofu until crispy. Blend cashews, almond milk, nutritional yeast, lemon juice, coconut aminos, turmeric, salt, and pepper until smooth. Pour the sauce into a skillet, heat it, and toss with spaghetti and tofu. Garnish with parsley.

**Servings-4, Kcal- 425**
**Proteins- 12g, Fats- 20g, Carbs- 48g**

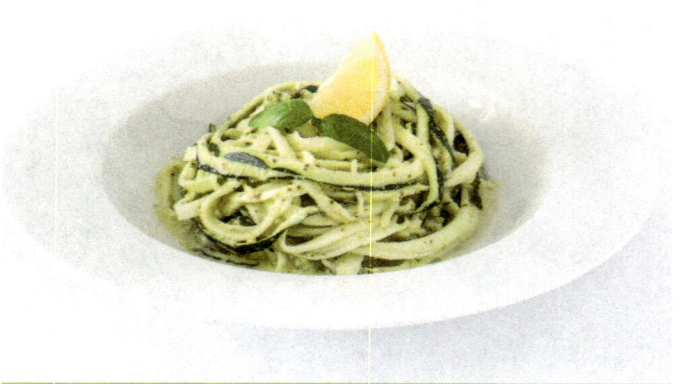

## Zucchini Noodle with Almond Butter

### Ingredients

- 1 cup zucchini noodles
- 2 tbsp almond butter
- 1 tbsp coconut aminos
- 1 tbsp lime juice
- 1 tsp honey
- Red pepper flakes

### Instructions

Toss zucchini noodles with a dressing made from almond butter, coconut aminos, lime juice, honey, and red pepper flakes.

**Servings-1, Kcal- 220**
**Proteins- 6g, Fats- 16g, Carbs- 14g**

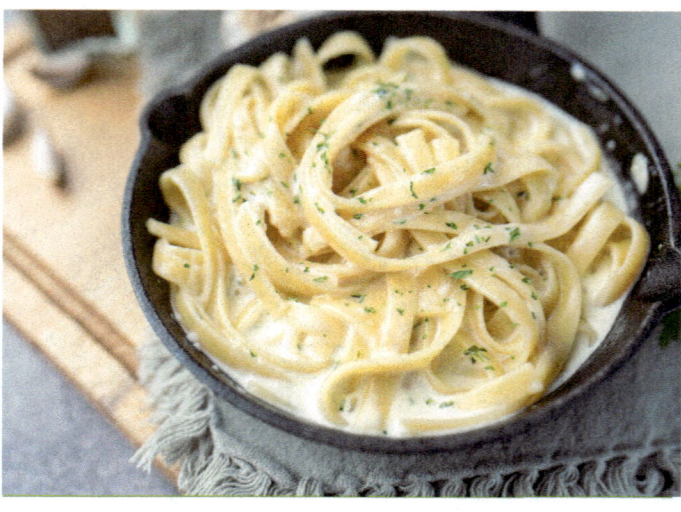

## Cashew Alfredo Pasta

### Ingredients

- 8 oz whole grain or chickpea pasta
- 1/2 cup raw cashews, soaked
- 1/2 cup water
- 2 tbsp nutritional yeast
- 1 tbsp lemon juice
- 1 garlic clove
- Salt and pepper to taste
- 1 tbsp olive oil
- Fresh parsley for garnish

### Instructions

Cook pasta according to package instructions. Drain. Blend soaked cashews, water, nutritional yeast, lemon juice, garlic, salt, and pepper until smooth. Heat olive oil in a pan, pour in the cashew sauce, and heat for 2-3 minutes. Toss cooked pasta in the sauce and garnish with parsley.

**Serving: 2, Calories: 350**
**Proteins: 10, Fats: 20, Carbs: 40**

# POULTRY

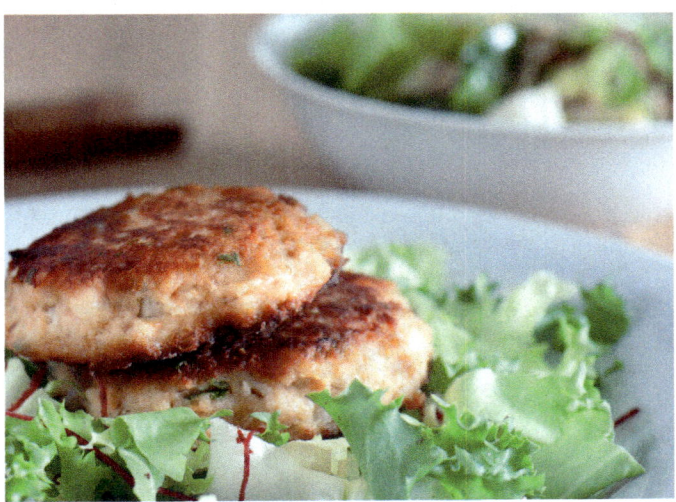

## Turkey Patties

### Ingredients

- 1 tablespoon olive oil
- ½ teaspoon sage
- Salt
- ¼ onion
- Pepper
- 3/4 pounds turkey(without skin)
- 1 egg

### Instructions

Mix Salt, Pepper, 1 egg, ½ teaspoon sage, ¼ onion, 3/4 pound turkey and form into 2 patties. In a frypan heat oil and add patties, cook well on both sides for 5-8 minutes.

**Servings-1, Kcal- 240**
**Proteins-65g, Fats- 36g, Carbs- 3g**

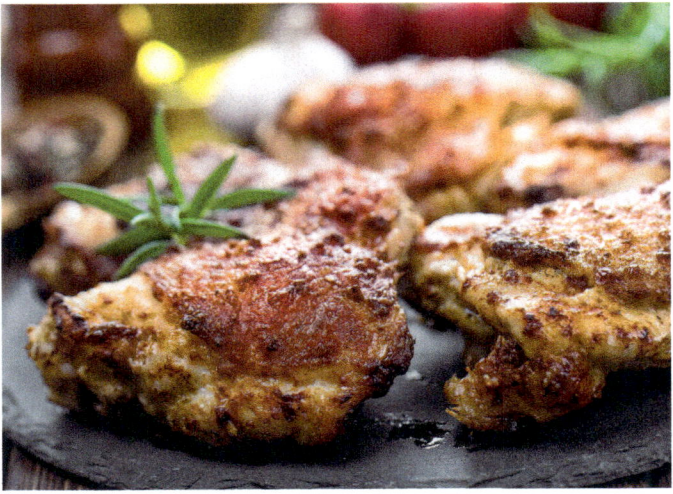

## Roasted chicken thighs

### Ingredients

- 2 pounds of boneless chicken thighs
- Ground pepper
- 1 tablespoon organic extra virgin olive oil
- Fresh cilantro
- 1 tablespoon chili powder
- Lime wedges
- Sea salt to taste

### Instructions

Preheat the oven to 140 degrees C. Place the chicken on a baking sheet. Drizzle with olive oil and turn to coat. Rub with chili powder, salt, and pepper. Roast the chicken legs in the oven for about 40 minutes. Sprinkle with coriander and serve with lime wedges. For the Air Fryer: Air fry at 375°F (190°C) for 18-20 minutes, flipping halfway.

**Servings-3, Kcal- 573**
**Proteins- 105g, Fats- 15g, Carbs- 2g**

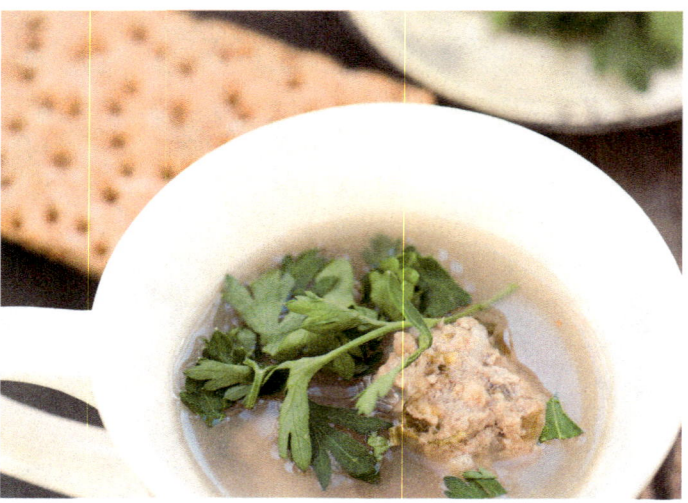
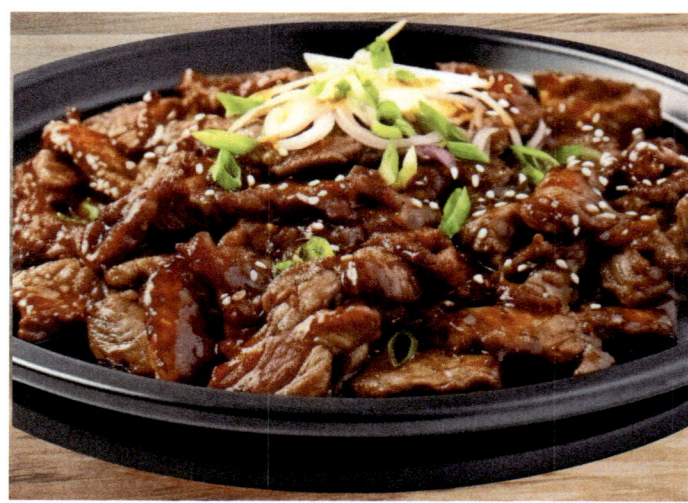

## Asian Soup with Chicken Meatballs

### Ingredients

**For chicken balls:** Salt and pepper
- 0.6 lb. chopped chicken (270 g)
- 1 tablespoon chives (3 g),
- 2 tablespoons of avocado oil
- 1 tablespoon fresh ginger finely

**For the broth:** Coriander
- 2.5 cups of chicken broth (600 ml)
- 2 green onions (10 g), sliced
- 1 teaspoon fish sauce (5 ml)
- 5 slices of fresh ginger (5 g)

### Instructions

Mix chicken with chives, ginger, salt, and pepper. Shape into ping-pong-sized balls and chill. Simmer broth with fish sauce and ginger for 10-15 minutes. Sear chicken balls in oil until golden and cooked through. Adjust broth seasoning, strain, and divide into bowls. Add meatballs, top with spring onions, and garnish with coriander.

**Servings-2, Kcal- 266**
**Proteins- 45g, Fats- 8g, Carbs- 4g**

## Chicken bulgogi

### Ingredients

- 3 tablespoons of avocado oil
- 1/2 tablespoon sesame oil
- 1 chicken breast, cut into thin strips
- 2 cloves of garlic, minced
- 1/2 medium onion, diced
- Salt, to taste
- 3 tablespoons coconut aminos
- 1 teaspoon sesame seeds

### Instructions

Heat avocado oil in a large pan over medium heat. Add chicken and onion to the pan and fry until the chicken is cooked (about 5-7 minutes). Add coconut aminos, sesame oil, and garlic to the pan and fry for about 1 minute. Season with salt and garnish with sesame seeds.

**Servings-1, Kcal- 650**
**Proteins- 50g, Fats- 30g, Carbs- 3g**

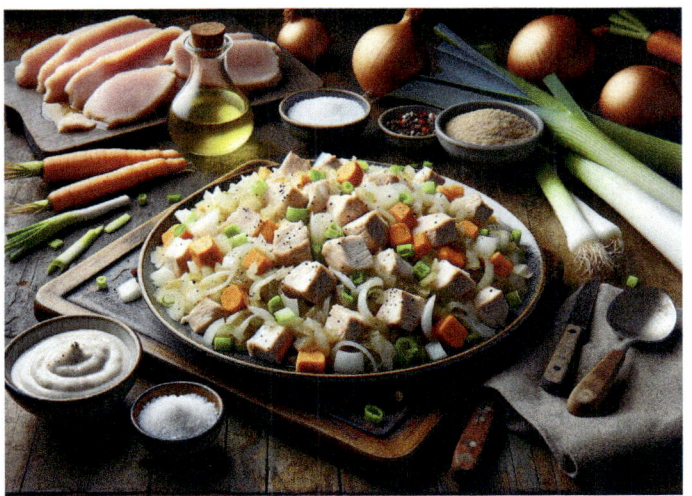

## Chicken Hash Recipe

### Ingredients

- 4 chicken breasts
- 1 leek, sliced
- 1 medium onion, sliced
- 4 tablespoons coconut oil
- 2 carrots, grated
- Salt and pepper, to taste
- Coconut Dijon sauce

### Instructions

Cook the diced chicken breast in coconut oil and fry until properly cooked. Season with salt and pepper as desired. If necessary, add more coconut oil to the pan and cook the vegetables gently. Add the chicken pieces back. Serve with Dijon coconut sauce.

**Servings-2, Kcal- 600**
**Proteins- 110g, Fats- 21g, Carbs- 3g**

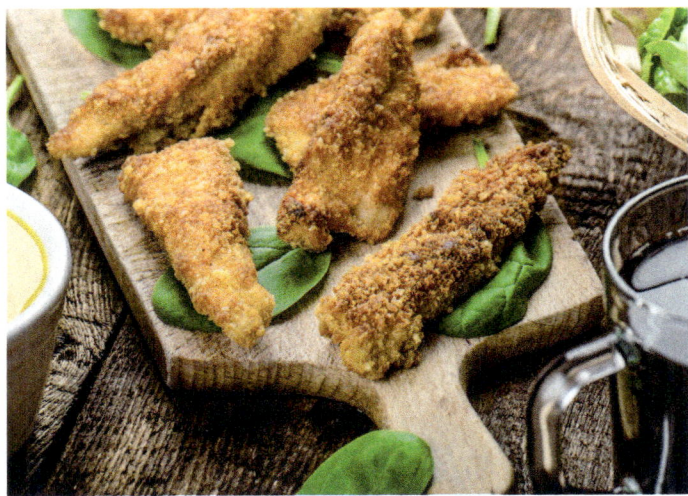

## Coconut Chicken Tenders

### Ingredients

- 1 pound boneless chicken
- 1/4 teaspoon salt
- 1 egg
- 1/4 teaspoon pepper
- 1/2 cup cashew flour
- 1/4 teaspoon garlic powder
- 1 cup unsweetened shredded coconut
- 1/8 teaspoon of cinnamon

### Instructions

Preheat the oven to 170 degrees C. Beat the egg in a bowl and set aside. Combine cashew flour, coconut, and spices in another bowl. Dip each chicken tender first in the egg and then in the batter. Place the coated chicken tenders on a baking sheet lined with aluminum foil or parchment paper. Bake for 25 to 30 minutes. For the Air Fryer: Air fry at 375°F (190°C) for 14-18 minutes.

**Servings-2, Kcal- 510**
**Proteins- 92g, Fats- 15g, Carbs- 7g**

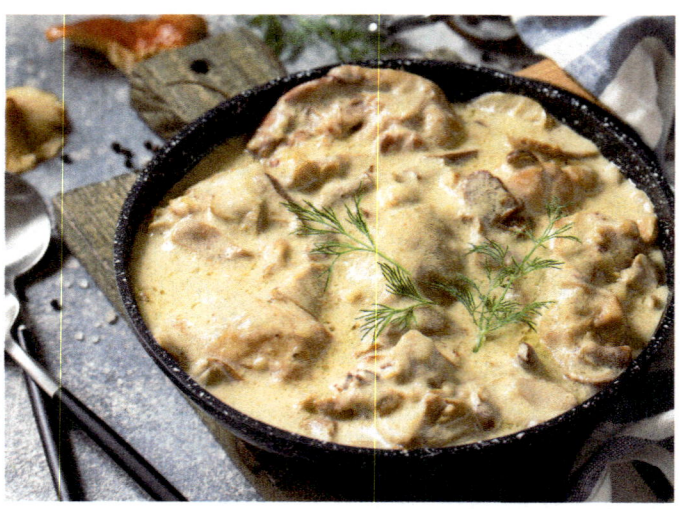

## Easy coconut chicken

### Ingredients

- 1 tablespoon coconut oil
- 1/2 teaspoon black pepper
- 5 cloves garlic
- 1/2 teaspoon Sea Salt
- 4 tablespoons of apple cider vinegar
- 1/4 cup water
- 1 lb boneless skinless, chicken thighs
- 1 cup coconut milk, canned

### Instructions

Add the chicken and coconut oil to a large pan over medium/low heat. Cook for 2-3 minutes. Add apple cider vinegar, water, and garlic; cook for 3 minutes. Add salt and pepper and cook until the liquid evaporates, about 10 minutes. Stir in coconut milk and simmer for 5-10 minutes until the sauce thickens. Enjoy!

**Servings-1, Kcal- 750**
**Proteins- 150g, Fats- 15g, Carbs- 4g**

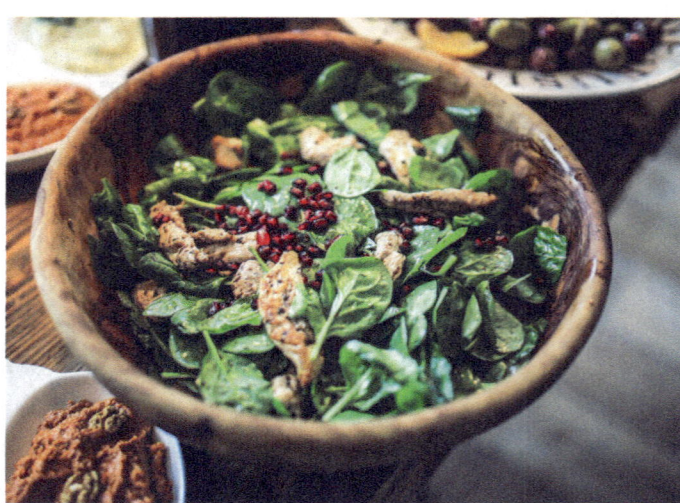

## Easy Chicken + Spinach

### Ingredients

- Cooked chicken breast: 2 cups, shredded or diced (about 300g)
- Fresh spinach: 4 cups (about 120g)
- Pomegranate seeds: 1 cup (about 150g)
- Optional dressing: 2 tablespoons olive oil, 1 tablespoon lemon juice, 1 teaspoon honey, and a pinch of salt and pepper

### Instructions

Combine the spinach, shredded chicken, and pomegranate seeds in a large bowl. If desired, whisk together the dressing ingredients and drizzle over the salad. Toss gently to combine and serve immediately.

**Servings-2, Kcal- 450**
**Proteins- 29g, Fats- 20g, Carbs- 18g**

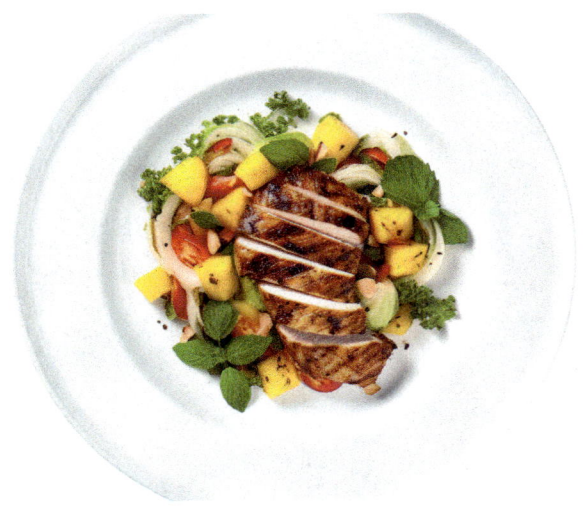

## Mango and Grilled Chicken Salad

### Ingredients

- Lime, juice of (1 lime)
- Honey (1 tablespoon)
- Avocado, sliced (1 ripe)
- Olive oil (2 tablespoons )
- Mixed salad greens (4 cups)
- Mango, diced (2 ripe mangos)
- Red onion, thinly sliced (1 small)
- Fresh cilantro, chopped (garnish)
- Cucumber, thinly sliced (1 medium)
- Sea salt and black pepper, to taste
- Chili flakes (1/4 teaspoon, optional)
- Toasted cashews or almonds (1/4 cup)
- Chicken breasts, grilled (2 medium)

### Instructions

Toss greens, mango, cucumber, onion, and avocado. Whisk olive oil, lime juice, honey, chili flakes (optional), salt, and pepper for dressing. Arrange salad, top with chicken, drizzle dressing, and garnish with cilantro and nuts.

**Servings-2, Kcal- 730**
**Proteins- 39g, Fats- 38g, Carbs- 66g**

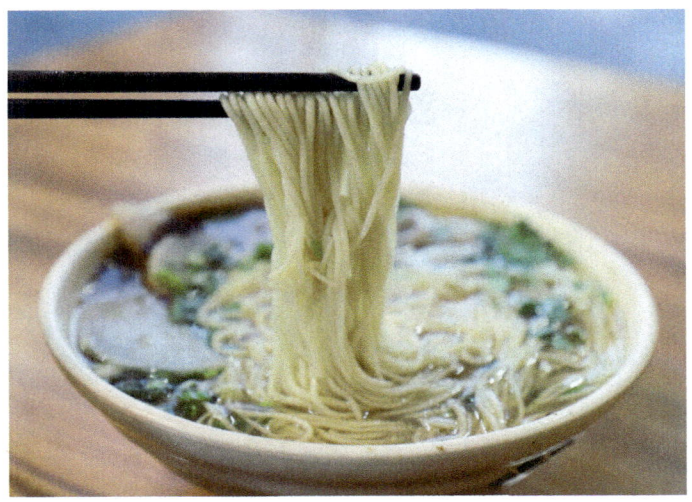

## Chayote Chicken Noodle Soup

### Ingredients

- 1 tablespoon olive oil
- 1 cup water
- 1/2 onion diced
- 1 teaspoon basil dried
- 6 cups of chicken broth
- 1 teaspoon oregano dried
- 1 pound chicken pre-cooked
- 1 teaspoon parsley dried
- Salt and pepper to taste
- 2 chayote squash

### Instructions

Heat oil in a large saucepan over medium heat. Cook onion and celery until translucent, about 5 minutes. Add broth, water, chicken, herbs, salt, and pepper. Boil, then simmer covered for 10 minutes. Spiralize chayote into noodles. Add to soup, simmer uncovered for 10 minutes.

**Servings-1, Kcal- 700**
**Proteins- 150g, Fats- 11g, Carbs- 5g**

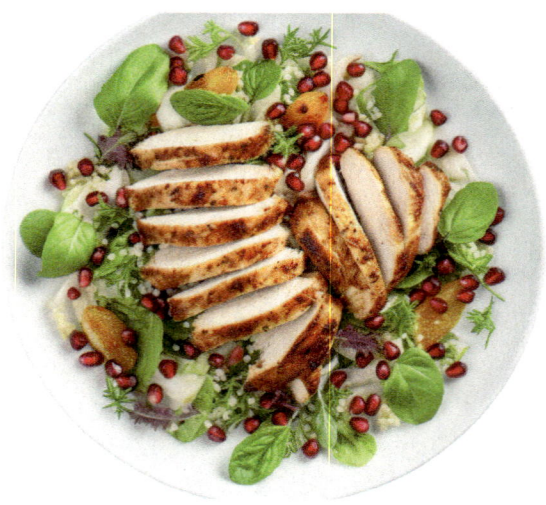

## Pomegranate Chicken Salad

### Ingredients

- Pomegranate seeds (from 1 fruit )
- Chicken breasts (2 medium-sized)
- Olive oil (3 tablespoons for dressing)
- Fresh rosemary, minced (1 teaspoon)
- Walnuts, chopped (1/2 cup optional)
- Red onion, thinly sliced (1 small)
- Sea salt and black pepper (to taste)
- Mixed salad greens (4 cups)
- Avocado, sliced (1 ripe)
- Lemon, juice of (1 lemon)
- Honey (1 tablespoon)

### Instructions

Season chicken with rosemary, salt, and pepper, then grill 6-7 minutes per side until 165°F (75°C). Let rest, then slice. Toss greens, pomegranate, walnuts, avocado, and onion. Whisk olive oil, honey, lemon juice, salt, and pepper for dressing. Plate the salad, top with chicken, drizzle with dressing.

**Servings-1, Kcal- 745**
**Proteins- 40g, Fats- 54g, Carbs- 35g**

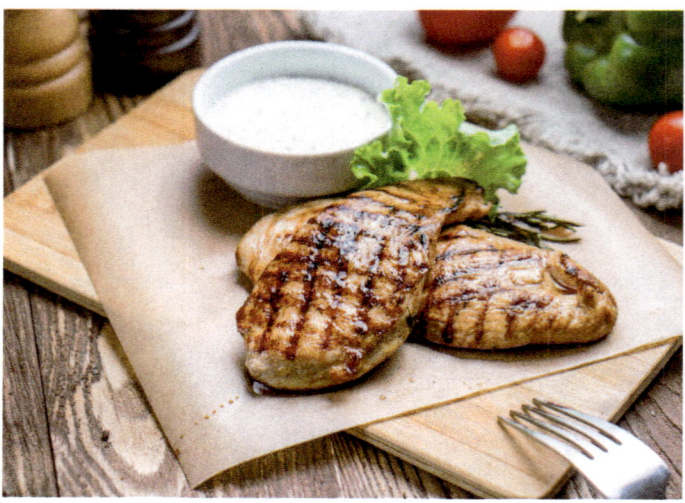

## Marinated Grilled Chicken

### Ingredients

- 1/4 cup balsamic vinegar
- 1-1/2 teaspoons lemon juice
- 2 tablespoons of olive oil
- 1/2 teaspoon lemon-pepper seasoning
- 4 boneless skinless chicken breast halves (6 ounces each)

### Instructions

Combine vinegar, oil, lemon juice, and lemon pepper in a large plastic bag, add chicken. Close the bag. Store in the refrigerator for 30 minutes. Drain and throw away the marinade. Moisten a paper towel with cooking oil; using long-handled tongs, lightly coat the grill rack. Grill over medium heat for 5-7 minutes per side or until the thermometer shows 170 °. For the oven, bake at 200°C (400°F) on a lined baking sheet for 20-25 minutes, flipping halfway, until a thermometer reads 170°C.

**Servings-3, Kcal- 400**
**Proteins- 75g, Fats- 12g, Carbs- 3g**

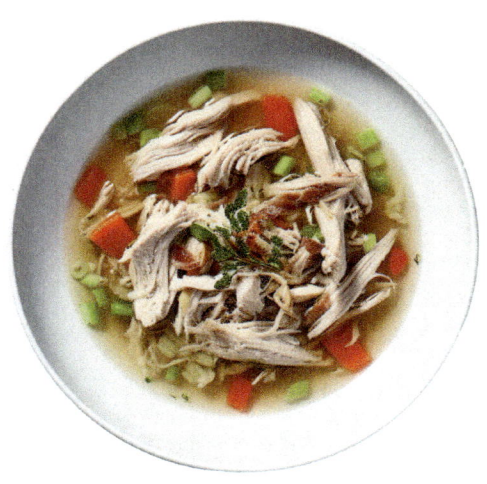
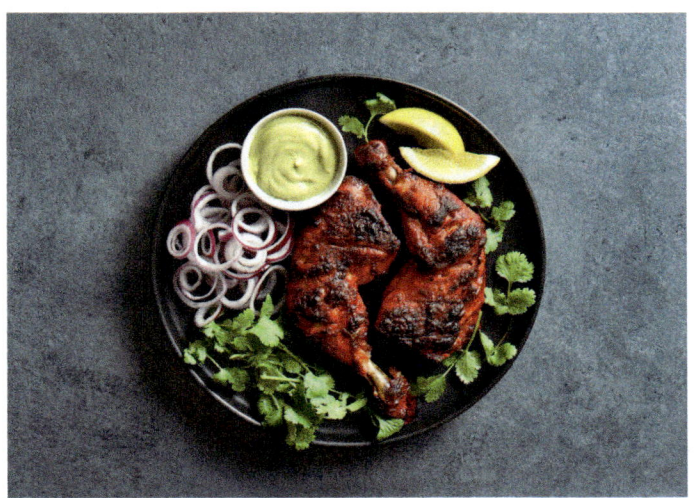

## Herbed Turkey and Vegetable Soup

### Ingredients

- Zucchini, Onion diced (1)
- Ground turkey (1 lb.)
- Juice of (1/2 a lemon)
- Olive oil (2 tablespoons)
- Garlic cloves, minced (3)
- Carrots, diced (2 medium)
- Dried thyme, Rosemary (2 tsp each)
- Celery stalks, chopped (2)
- Dried oregano (1 teaspoon)
- Green beans, chopped (1 cup)
- Turmeric powder (1/2 teaspoon)
- Sea salt and black pepper, to taste
- Chicken or vegetable broth (8 cups )

### Instructions

Sauté onions, garlic, carrots, and celery for 5 minutes. Add turkey and cook until browned. Stir in green beans, zucchini, herbs, and turmeric. Pour in broth, bring to a boil, and simmer for 20-25 minutes. Season with salt, pepper, and lemon juice.

**Servings - 2, Calories: 650**
**Carbs: 22 g | Fat: 37 g |Protein: 54 g**

## Jamaican Chicken Fajitas

### Ingredients

- Olive oil (1 tbsp.)
- Pepper and salt (as desired)
- Chicken legs (2)
- Lime (1)
- Taco seasoning (1 t.)
- Sliced red onion (0.25 cup)

### Instructions

Preheat the oven to 400°F (200°C). In a mixing bowl, toss the chicken legs with seasonings and oil. Arrange them on a lined baking sheet in a single layer. Bake for 40-45 minutes, flipping halfway, until the internal temperature reaches 165°F (74°C). Serve with cilantro and lime juice. For the Air Fryer: Air fry at 390°F (199°C) for 25-30 minutes, flipping halfway, until the chicken reaches 165°F (74°C).

**Servings - 2, Calories: 386**
**Carbs: 6 g | Fat: 30 g | Protein: 25 g**

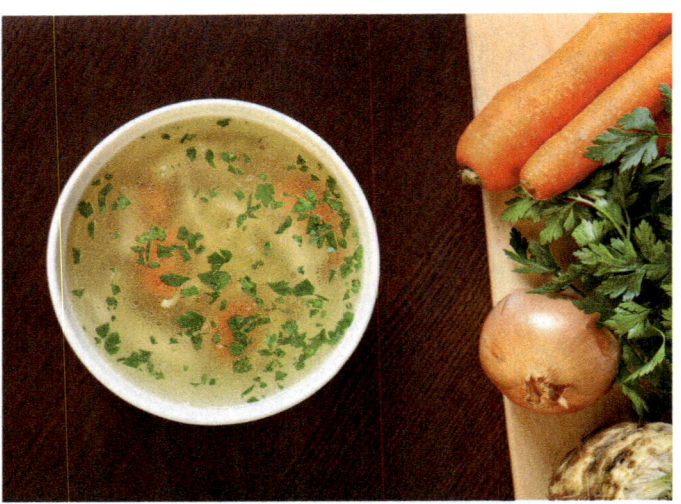

## Chicken Soup

### Ingredients

- 1 whole chicken
- 2 tablespoons Italian spice
- 5 chopped celery stalks
- 2 liters of water
- 2 medium carrots, chopped
- 2 tablespoons of salt
- 1 medium onion, chopped
- 1 teaspoon black pepper
- 3 garlic cloves, peeled and chopped
- 1/4 cup parsley chopped

### Instructions

Combine chicken, Italian spice, celery, water, carrots, salt, onion, pepper, and garlic in a large pot. Boil, then simmer covered for 1.5–2 hours, skimming foam. Remove chicken, shred, discard bones, and return meat to the pot. Simmer for 10 more minutes, garnish with parsley, and serve hot.

**Servings-6, Kcal- 275**
**Proteins- 57g, Fats- 4g, Carbs- 3g**

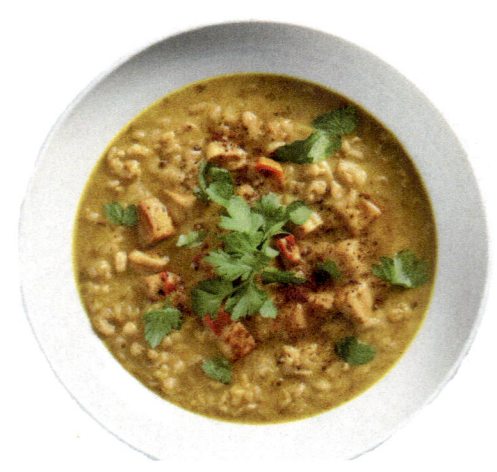

## Curried Lentil Chicken Soup

### Ingredients

- Chicken breasts diced (1 lb. boneless )
- Lentils rinsed (1 cup green or brown)
- Olive oil or coconut oil (2 tbsp)
- Chili powder (1/4 teaspoon optional)
- Chicken broth (8 cups low-sodium)
- Sea salt and black pepper, to taste
- Curry powder (2 teaspoons)
- Cilantro, chopped (garnish)
- Celery stalks, chopped (2)
- Garlic cloves , minced (3)
- Onion,Carrot diced (1 each)
- Turmeric (1 teaspoon)
- Cumin (1/2 teaspoon)
- Juice of (1 lemon)

### Instructions

Heat oil in a pot over medium heat. Sauté onions, garlic, carrots, and celery for 5 minutes. Add chicken and cook for 4-6 minutes. Stir in spices, coating well. Add broth and lentils, boil, then simmer for 25-30 minutes—season with salt, pepper, and lemon juice. Garnish with cilantro.

**Servings - 2, Calories: 700**
**Protein: 85 g | Carbs: 36 g | Fat: 25 g**

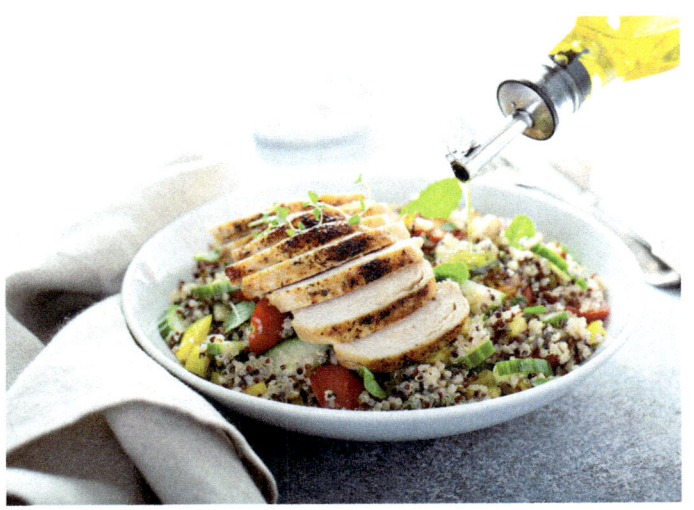 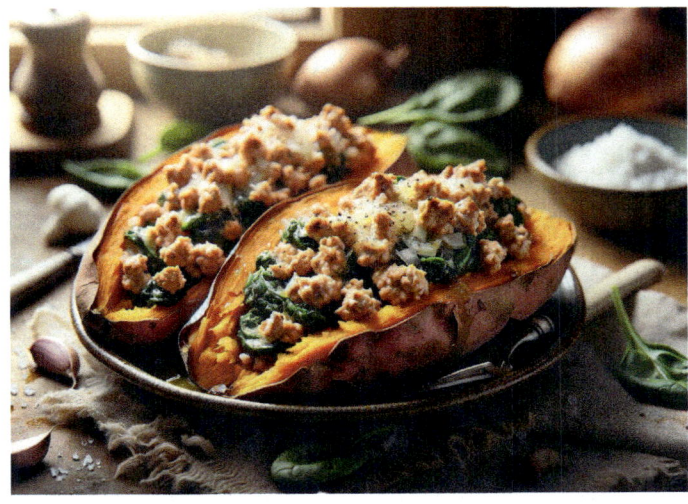

## Grilled Chicken and Quinoa Salad

### Ingredients

- 1 large chicken breast (about 200g)
- 1/2 cup (90g) quinoa
- 3 cups (90g) mixed greens
- 1/2 cup (50g) cucumber, sliced
- 2 tbsp (30ml) olive oil
- 1 tbsp (15ml) lemon juice
- Salt and pepper to taste

### Instructions

Grill the chicken breast and season with salt and pepper. Cook quinoa as per the package instructions. Toss mixed greens, and sliced cucumber with cooked quinoa, olive oil, and lemon juice. Slice the grilled chicken and serve on top of the salad.

**Serving: 2, Calories: 420**
**Proteins: 27, Fats: 23, Carbs: 27**

## Turkey and Spinach Sweet Potatoes

### Ingredients

- 2 medium sweet potatoes
- 200g ground turkey
- 1 cup (30g) spinach, chopped
- 1/2 small onion (50g), diced
- 2 cloves garlic, minced
- 1 tbsp (15ml) olive oil
- Salt and pepper to taste

### Instructions

Bake sweet potatoes at 400°F (200°C) for 40-50 minutes until tender. Sauté onion and garlic in olive oil, add turkey and cook until browned. Stir in spinach, season, and cook until wilted. Slice sweet potatoes and fluff, and fill with turkey mixture. For Air Fryer: Air fry at 400°F (200°C) for 35-40 minutes.

**Serving: 2, Calories: 451**
**Proteins: 27, Fats: 16, Carbs: 44**

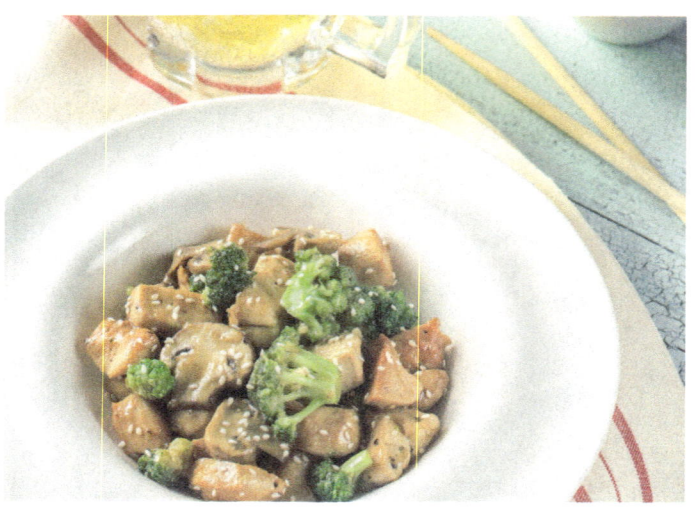

## Chicken and Broccoli Stir-Fry

### Ingredients

- 1 lb chicken breast
- 1 head of broccoli
- 2 garlic cloves
- Coconut aminos
- Honey
- Sesame oil
- Olive oil
- Sesame seeds

### Instructions

Dice chicken and broccoli. Sauté in olive oil until chicken browns. Add garlic and broccoli; cook until vibrant. Combine coconut amino, honey, sesame oil; add to pan. Coat well; cook briefly. Garnish with sesame seeds.

**Serving: 4, Calories: 270**
**Proteins: 26, Fats: 12, Carbs: 13**

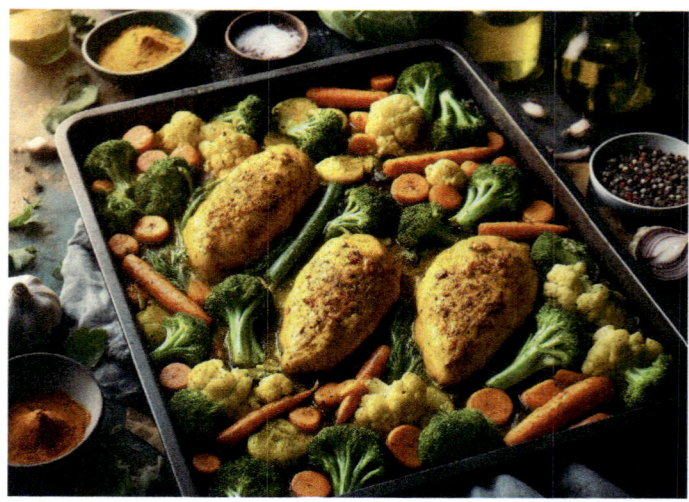

## Turmeric Chicken with Vegetables

### Ingredients

- 2 chicken breasts, diced
- 1 tbsp avocado oil
- 1 tsp turmeric
- Black pepper, sea salt ( 1/2 tsp each)
- 2 cloves garlic, minced
- Broccoli, carrots, zucchini ( 1 cup each)
- 1 tbsp lemon juice
- 1/2 tsp ground cumin
- 1/4 tsp chili flakes (optional)
- Fresh cilantro for garnish

### Instructions

Heat avocado oil in a skillet over medium heat. Add diced chicken, turmeric, black pepper, and salt. Sauté until chicken is golden and cooked through (about 5-7 minutes). Stir in garlic, cumin, and chili flakes, cooking for another minute. Add broccoli, carrots, and zucchini. Sauté for 5 minutes until veggies are tender but still crisp. Drizzle with lemon juice and mix well. Garnish with fresh cilantro.

**Serving: 2, Calories: 310**
**Proteins: 35, Fats: 11, Carbs: 16**

# DESSERTS

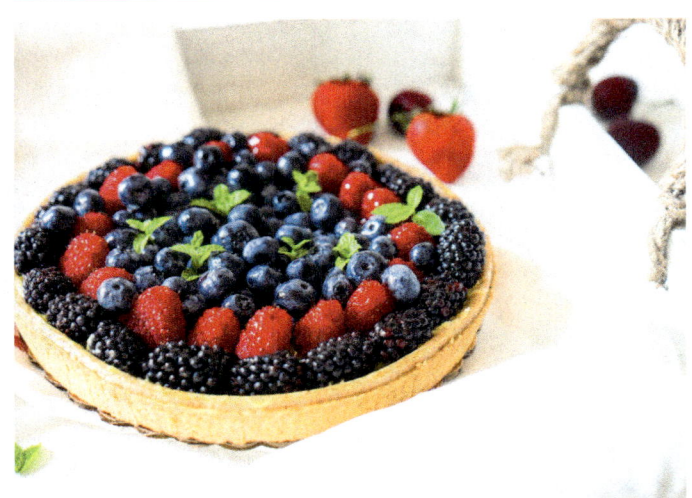

## Summer Berry Tart

### Ingredients

**For the crust –**
- 1 1/2 cups almond flour
- 1/4 cup coconut oil
- 1/4 cup maple syrup

**For the filling –**
- 1 cup cashews (soaked)
- 1/2 cup coconut cream
- 1/4 cup maple syrup
- 2 cups mixed berries

### Instructions

Preheat oven to 350°F (175°C). Mix almond flour, melted coconut oil, and maple syrup, press into a tart pan, and bake for 12-15 minutes. Blend cashews, coconut cream, and maple syrup until smooth for the filling. Pour into the cooled crust and chill. Top with fresh berries before serving. For Air Fryer: Air fry at 175°C (350°F) for 10-12 minutes.

**Serving: 8, Calories: 35**
**Proteins: 7, Fats: 27, Carbs: 25**

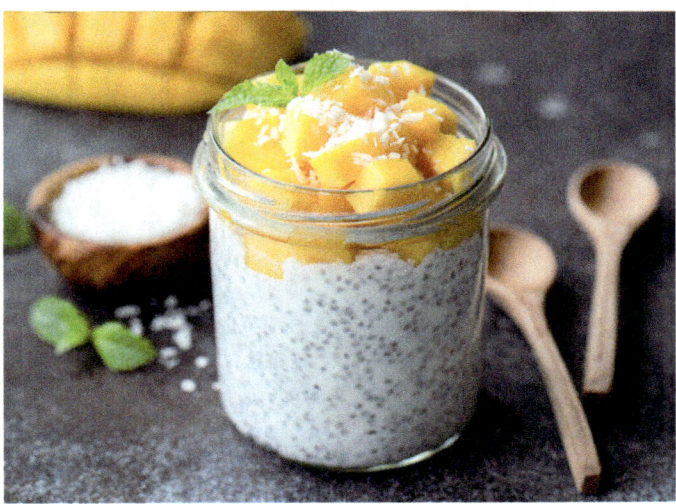

## Green Tea Chia Pudding

### Ingredients

- 1/4 cup chia seeds
- 1 cup brewed green tea
- 1 tbsp maple syrup
- 1/2 tsp vanilla extract
- 1/4 cup diced mango
- 1 tbsp shredded coconut

### Instructions

Combine chia seeds with green tea, maple syrup, and vanilla extract. Stir well and let it sit overnight in the fridge. In the morning, top with diced mango and shredded coconut.

**Serving: 1, Calories: 256**
**Proteins: 5, Fats: 12, Carbs: 33**

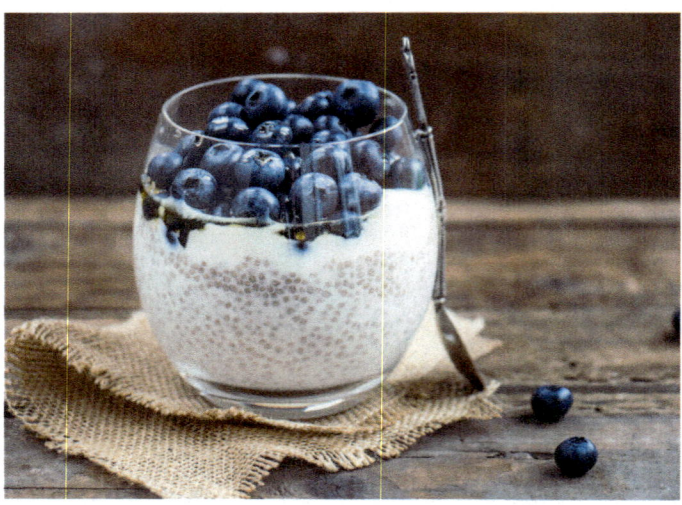

## Chia Seed and Blueberry Pudding

### Ingredients

- Sea salt (a pinch)
- Chia seeds (1/2 cup)
- Lemon zest (from 1 lemon)
- Vanilla extract (1 teaspoon)
- Blueberries (2 cups, fresh or frozen)
- Almond milk or coconut milk (2 cups)
- Maple syrup (1/4 cup, adjust to taste)

### Instructions

Mix chia seeds, maple syrup, almond or coconut milk, vanilla, and sea salt in a bowl—Refrigerate for 4 hours or overnight until gel-like. Blend 1.5 cups blueberries until smooth, adding maple syrup if desired. Stir lemon zest into the pudding, then layer or mix with blueberry puree. Serve topped with remaining blueberries.

**Serving: 4, Calories: 185**
**Proteins: 4, Fats: 8, Carbs: 23**

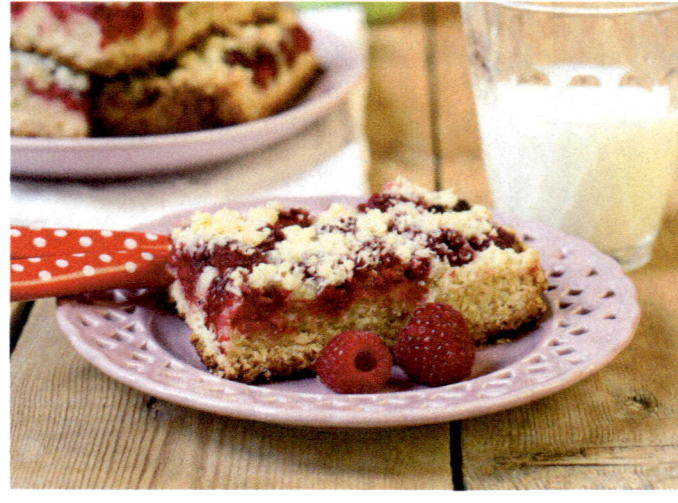

## Raspberry Coconut Bars

### Ingredients

- 1 1/2 cups almond flour
- 1/4 cup honey
- 1/4 cup melted coconut oil
- 1 cup fresh raspberries
- 1/2 cup coconut flakes

### Instructions

Preheat the oven to 350°F (175°C) and line an 8x8-inch baking dish with parchment paper. Combine 1 1/2 cups almond flour, 1/4 cup honey, and 1/4 cup melted coconut oil to form a dough. Press into the dish, top with 1 cup raspberries and 1/2 cup coconut flakes, and bake for 20-25 minutes until golden brown. Cool, cut into squares, and enjoy. For Air Fryer: Air fry at 320°F (160°C) for 15-18 minutes until golden brown.

**Serving: 12, Calories: 140**
**Proteins: 2, Fats: 10, Carbs: 12**

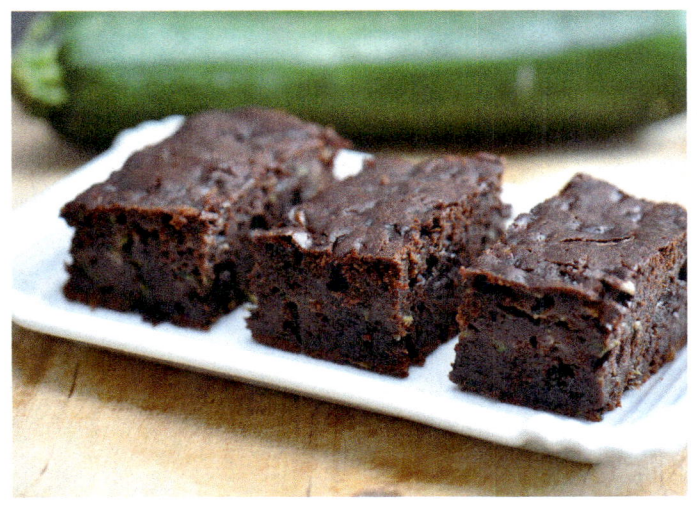

## Zucchini Brownies

### Ingredients

- 1 1/2 cups grated zucchini
- 1 cup almond flour
- 1/2 cup unsweetened cocoa powder
- 2 large eggs
- 1/2 cup honey

### Instructions

Preheat your oven to 350°F (175°C) and line an 8x8 inch baking dish. Mix 1 cup almond flour and 1/2 cup cocoa powder in a bowl. Whisk two eggs and 1/2 cup honey in another bowl. Combine wet and dry ingredients, then fold in 1 1/2 cups grated zucchini. Pour into the dish and bake for 25-30 minutes, until a toothpick comes out clean. Cool completely before cutting into squares. For Air Fryer: Air fry at 320°F (160°C) for 18-22 minutes until a toothpick comes out clean.

**Serving: 12, Calories: 110**
**Proteins: 3, Fats: 6, Carbs: 13**

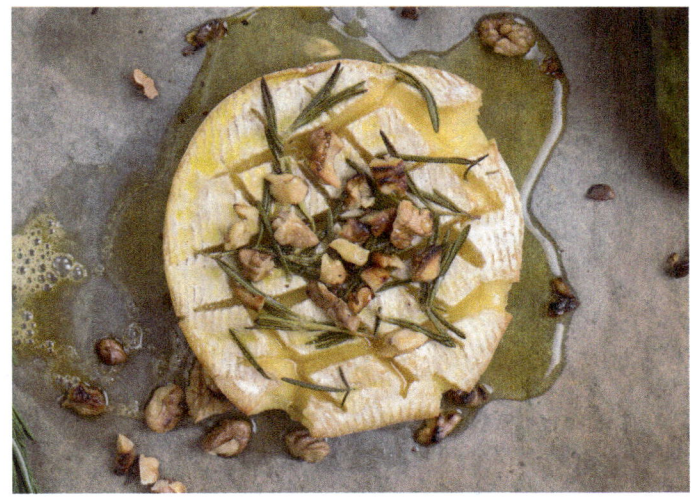

## Baked Pears with Walnuts and Honey

### Ingredients

- Pears: 1 medium pear
- Walnuts: 2 tablespoons (chopped)
- Honey: 1 tablespoon
- Cinnamon: 1/4 teaspoon

### Instructions

Preheat your oven to 350°F (175°C). Halve and core a pear, placing the halves in a baking dish cut side up. Sprinkle with 2 tablespoons of chopped walnuts and drizzle with 1 tablespoon of honey. Add a pinch of cinnamon. Bake for 20-25 minutes until tender. Let cool slightly before serving. For Air Fryer: Air fry at 350°F (175°C) for 12-15 minutes until tender.

**Serving: 1, Calories: 120**
**Proteins: 1, Fats: 5, Carbs: 20**

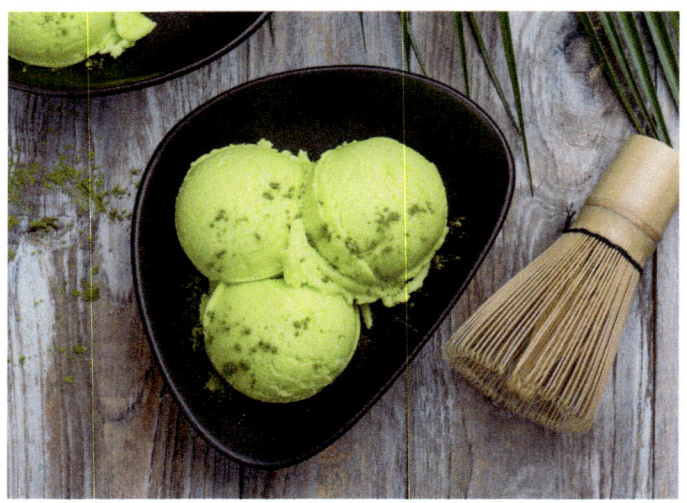

## Matcha Green Tea Ice Cream

### Ingredients

- Coconut milk: 1/2 cup
- Honey: 1 teaspoon
- Matcha green tea powder: 1/2 teaspoon
- Vanilla extract: 1/4 teaspoon

### Instructions

Whisk together coconut milk, sweetener, matcha, and vanilla. Freeze.

**Serving: 1, Calories: 200**
**Proteins: 2, Fats: 15, Carbs: 15**

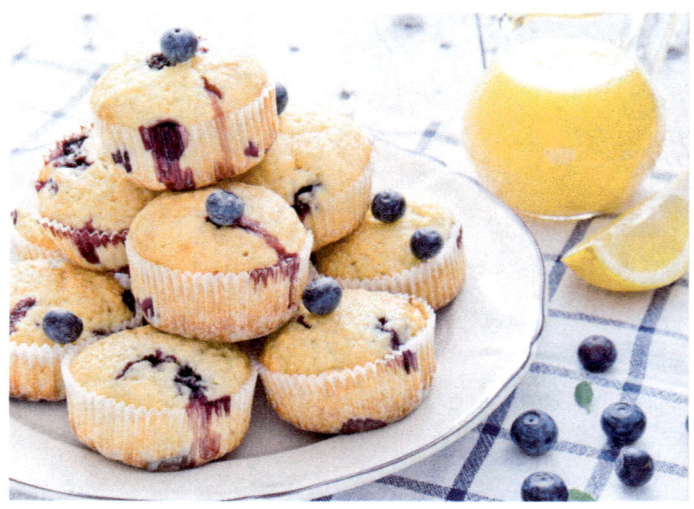

## Blueberry and Lemon Muffins

### Ingredients

- Almond flour: 3 tablespoons
- Eggs: 1 small egg
- Honey: 1 teaspoon
- Blueberries: 2 tablespoons
- Lemon zest: 1/4 teaspoon
- Baking powder: 1/8 teaspoon

### Instructions

Preheat the oven to 350°F (175°C). In a mixing bowl, combine 3 tablespoons almond flour, 1 small egg, 1 teaspoon honey, 2 tablespoons blueberries, 1/4 teaspoon lemon zest, and 1/8 teaspoon baking powder. Mix until well combined. Pour the batter into a greased or parchment-lined baking dish. Bake for 15-20 minutes or until a toothpick comes out clean. Let cool before serving. Enjoy! For the air fryer: Air fry at 350°F (175°C) for 10-12 minutes, or until golden and cooked through.

**Serving: 1, Calories: 140**
**Proteins: 5, Fats: 10, Carbs: 11**

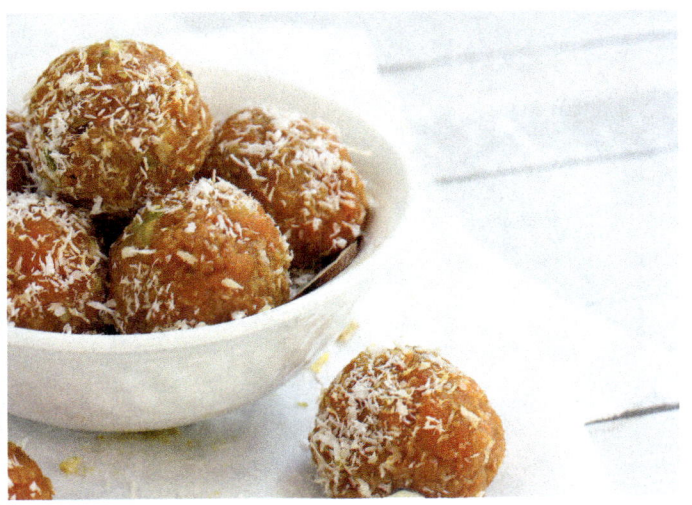

## Carrot Cake Bites

### Ingredients

- Grated carrot: 2 tablespoons
- Dates: 2 pitted dates
- Walnuts: 1 tablespoon (chopped)
- Coconut: 1 tablespoon (shredded)
- Cinnamon: 1/8 teaspoon

### Instructions

Process carrots, dates, walnuts, and cinnamon. Roll into balls and coat with coconut

**Serving: 1, Calories: 90**
**Proteins: 1, Fats: 5, Carbs: 11**

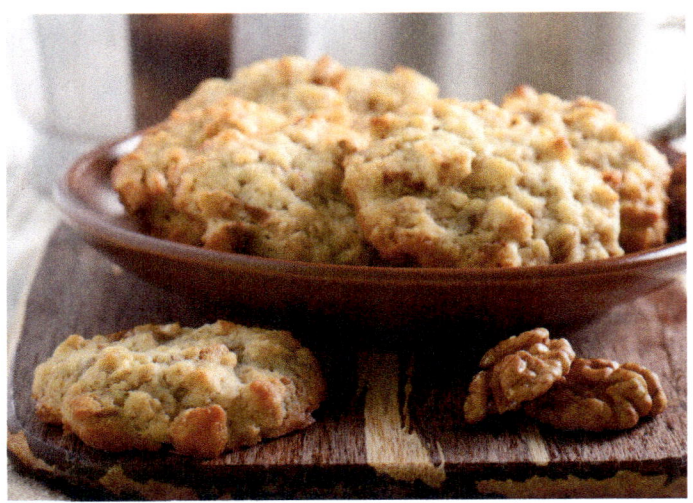

## Walnut and Oat Clusters

### Ingredients

- Walnuts: 2 tablespoons (chopped)
- Oats: 2 tablespoons
- Honey: 1 teaspoon
- Cinnamon: 1/8 teaspoon
- Vanilla extract: 1/4 teaspoon

### Instructions

Preheat the oven to 350°F (175°C). Combine walnuts, oats, honey, cinnamon, and vanilla in a mixing bowl. Stir well to coat the ingredients evenly. Spread the mixture onto a baking sheet in a single layer. Bake for 12-15 minutes, stirring halfway through, until the mixture is golden brown and crispy. Let it cool before serving. Enjoy! For Air fryer: Air fry at 350°F (175°C) for 8-10 minutes, stirring halfway through, until golden and crispy.

**Serving: 1, Calories: 160**
**Proteins: 4, Fats: 9, Carbs: 18**

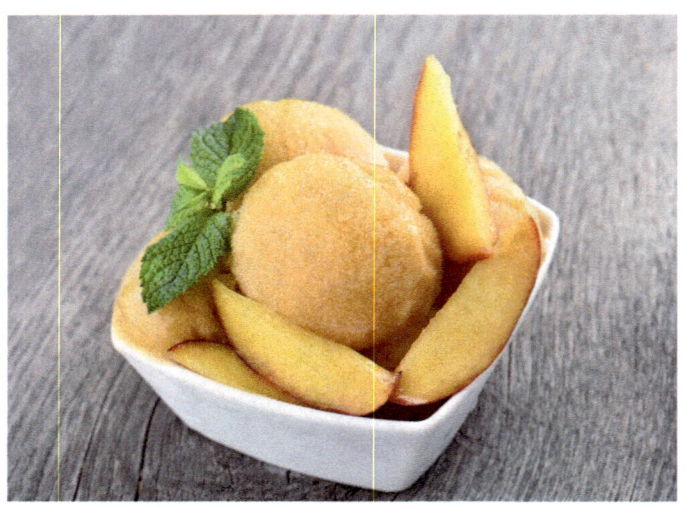

### Ginger Peach Sorbet

**Ingredients**

- Fresh peaches: 1 medium peach (peeled, pitted, and chopped)
- Grated ginger: 1/4 teaspoon
- Honey: 1 teaspoon
- Water: 1/4 cup

**Instructions**

Blend peaches, ginger, honey, and water until smooth. Freeze until set.

**Serving: 1, Calories: 100**
**Proteins: 1, Fats: 0, Carbs: 25**

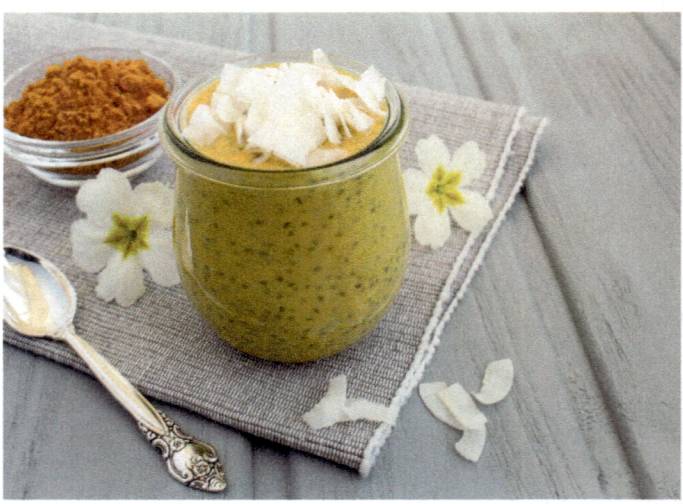

### Coconut Turmeric Chia Pudding

**Ingredients**

- Chia seeds: 2 tablespoons
- Coconut milk: 1/2 cup
- Turmeric: 1/4 teaspoon
- Honey: 1 teaspoon
- Vanilla extract: 1/4 teaspoon

**Instructions**

Mix chia seeds, coconut milk, turmeric, sweetener, and vanilla. Refrigerate overnight.

**Serving: 1, Calories: 180**
**Proteins: 3, Fats: 12, Carbs: 15**

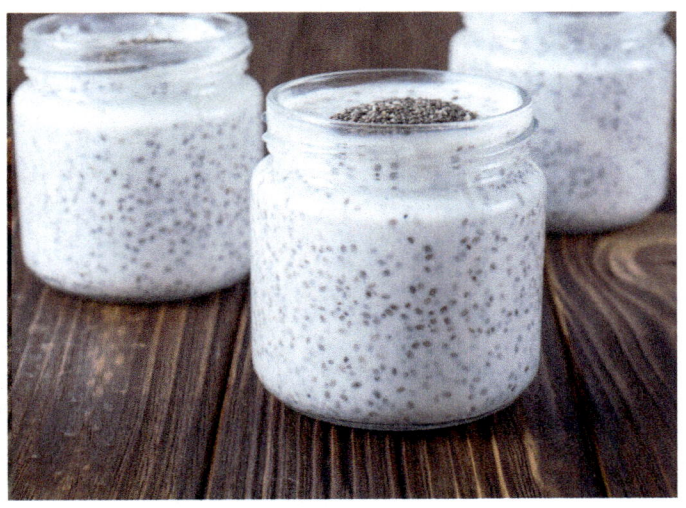

## Chia Seed Pudding

### Ingredients

- 1/4 cup chia seeds
- 1 cup almond milk
- 1 tbsp honey or maple syrup
- 1/2 tsp vanilla extract

### Instructions

Mix all ingredients in a bowl and let sit for 30 minutes or until it gets into a pudding consistency. Stir occasionally to prevent clumping. Serve with fresh fruit or a sprinkle of cinnamon.

**Servings - 2, Calories: 150**
**Proteins: 4, Fats: 8, Carbs: 16**

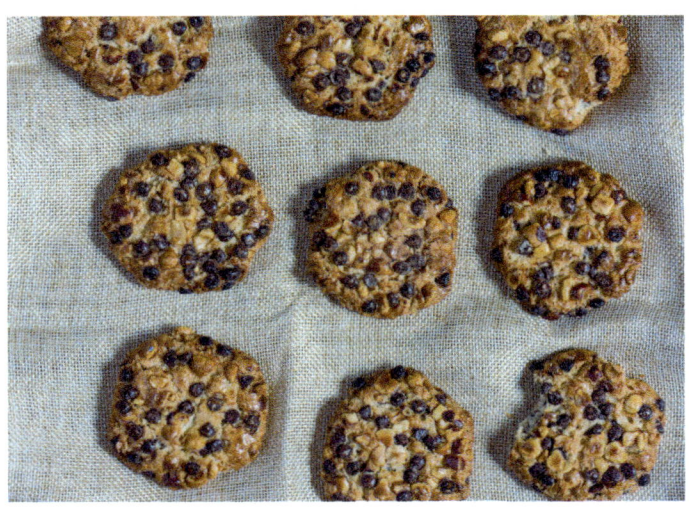

## Oatmeal and Banana Cookies

### Ingredients

- 2 ripe bananas, mashed
- 1 cup rolled oats
- 1/4 cup dark chocolate chips
- 1/2 tsp cinnamon

### Instructions

Preheat oven to 350°F (175°C). Mix all ingredients in a bowl. Spoon onto a baking sheet and shape into cookies. Bake for 15 minutes or until the edges are golden. For Air Fryer: Air fry at 350°F (175°C) for 8-10 minutes, flipping halfway, until the edges are golden.

**Servings - 12, Calories: 80**
**Proteins: 2, Fats: 3, Carbs: 18**

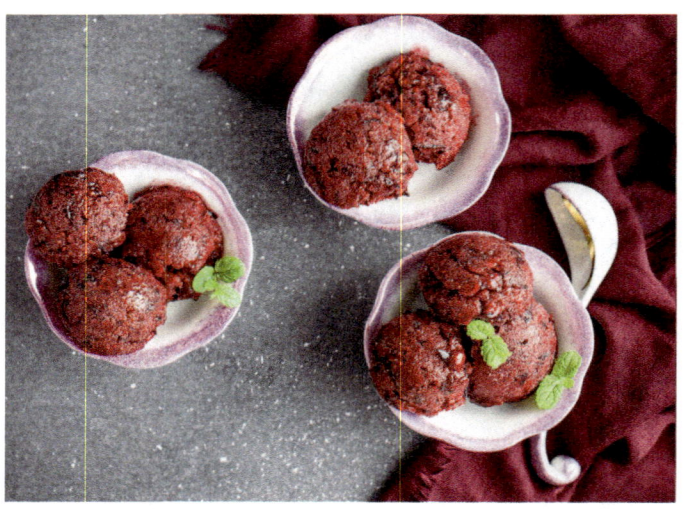

## Berry Sorbet

### Ingredients

- 4 cups frozen mixed berries
- Juice of one lemon
- 1/4 cup honey or maple syrup

### Instructions

Blend berries, sweetener, and lemon juice until smooth. Freeze in an airtight container for about 1 hour, stirring every 20 minutes, until it reaches a sorbet-like consistency.

**Serving: 4, Calories: 120**
**Proteins: 2, Fats: 1, Carbs: 35**

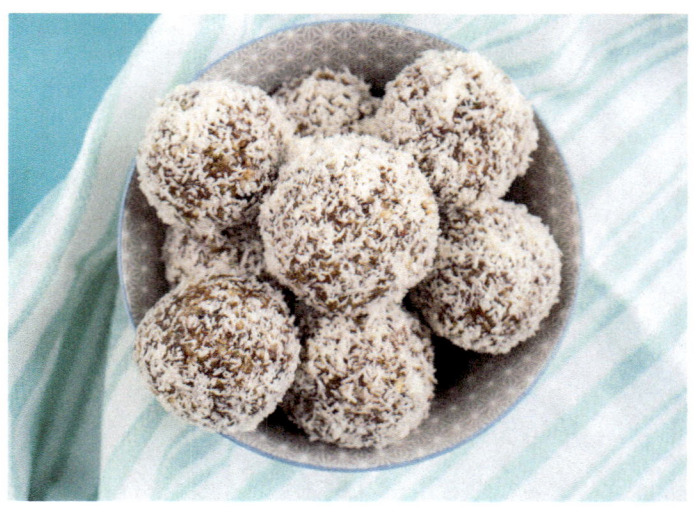

## Almond and Date Truffles

### Ingredients

- 1 cup dates (pitted)
- 1 cup almonds
- 1/4 cup cocoa powder
- 1 tsp vanilla extract
- Desiccated coconut for coating

### Instructions

Process dates and almonds in a food processor until they form a sticky mixture. Add cocoa powder and vanilla, and process again. Roll into balls and coat with desiccated coconut. Chill before serving.

**Serving: 12, Calories: 100**
**Proteins: 3, Fats: 4, Carbs: 12**

## Thank You for Completing this book!

We hope this book has inspired you to embrace more healthy meals daily. Your support means the world to us, and now that you've explored all the recipes, we'd love to hear your thoughts!

## Did you enjoy the book?

Please consider sharing your experience by leaving a review. Your feedback helps us improve and guides others on their journey toward healthier, more sustainable eating.

## Share Your Review

Your words could encourage someone to start their own plant-based adventure. Thank you for helping us spread the joy of plant-based living!

**We Value Your Feedback – Share Your Experience!**

Thank you for choosing the Anti-Inflammatory Cookbook for Easy Recipes. We hope this cookbook has been a valuable resource on your journey to a healthier lifestyle. Every recipe, tip, and meal plan was crafted with your success in mind, and we genuinely hope you've enjoyed exploring the delicious possibilities of the Anti-Inflammatory diet.

We value your experience and satisfaction. If this book has helped you simplify your cooking, introduced you to new flavors, or made your health journey more enjoyable, we would be thrilled if you could take a few moments to share your thoughts in a review. Whether it's a favorite recipe, the convenience of the meal plan, or any other aspect you appreciated, your feedback will help us improve our future work and guide others to consider embracing this way of eating.

Leaving a review is quick and easy. Scan the barcode below, and you'll be taken directly to the review page. Your insights and experiences are invaluable to us and to the community of readers who, like you, are seeking to make the most of their health journey.

Thank you for being a part of our community and for allowing us to be part of your culinary adventures. Your support and feedback make it all possible. Happy cooking, and may your meals continue to be as nourishing and delicious as ever!

## About the Author

Rocky Hansen is a dedicated health advocate, researcher, and author specializing in anti-inflammatory nutrition and holistic wellness. With a passion for helping others achieve optimal health through natural means, Rocky has spent years studying the science behind inflammation and its impact on the body.

Combining his extensive knowledge with a love for cooking, Rocky has crafted a comprehensive guide and cookbook that educates and inspires readers to take control of their health through delicious and scientifically-backed recipes.

When he's not writing or experimenting in the kitchen, Rocky enjoys hiking, yoga, and exploring new health trends. He is committed to empowering others with the tools and information they need to lead healthier, more vibrant lives.

Printed in Dunstable, United Kingdom